Mental Health for Primary Care
A practical guide for non-specialists

Mental Health for Primary Care

A practical guide for non-specialists

MARK MORRIS

General Practitioner,
Falmouth, Cornwall

Foreword by
ANDREW POLMEAR

Senior Research Fellow
Academic Unit of Primary Care
University of Sussex

Radcliffe Publishing
Oxford • New York

Radcliffe Publishing Ltd
18 Marcham Road
Abingdon
Oxon OX14 1AA
United Kingdom

www.radcliffe-oxford.com

Electronic catalogue and worldwide online ordering facility.

British Library Cataloguing in Publication Data

A catalogue record for this book is available from the British Library.

ISBN-13: 978 184619 271 5

Typeset by Pindar NZ, Auckland, New Zealand
Printed and bound by TJI Digital, Padstow, Cornwall, UK

Contents

Foreword

Books on clinical management tend to fall into two groups. The majority describe management as though it exists as an entity in its own right; they present the information and leave it to clinicians to extract the relevant material and apply it, often learning the practicalities of the job by trial and error. There is, however, a minority of books that revel in those practicalities. They start with the patient and his or her problems and guide the reader step-by-step through the consultation, showing through examples exactly how it can be done.

Mark Morris has written a book that is firmly in the latter group. He does discuss theoretical considerations but only enough for the reader to understand what is to follow; and he does it with a lightness of touch that makes them a joy to read. He then takes the reader through a series of consultations that cover the bulk of mental health problems in primary care. He gives examples of what to say and how to say it, conveying the excitement one has when one sits in with a skilled practitioner. By the end of the book the reader has been taken on a tour of the main psychotherapeutic interventions that are feasible in general practice, and will understand how cognitive behavioural therapy, non-directional counselling and an array of other approaches can be used by a busy general practitioner.

I longed for a book like this when I was in clinical practice. I am very pleased to find that it has been written at last and written so well.

Andrew Polmear MA MSc FRCP FRCGP
Former General Practitioner and Senior Research Fellow,
Academic Unit of Primary Care, The Trafford Centre,
University of Sussex
September 2008

Preface

Much of the available psychiatric literature is written by experts in the specialist setting. It mainly targets the specialist practitioner. There is an emphasis on illness and disorder rather than on mental health and its relationship to health overall: on well defined conditions rather than the 'emerging' poorly defined problems that are seen by most health practitioners. People seek help in primary care with varying degrees of distress and dysfunction. Presenting problems in primary care, where 90% of mental health difficulty is treated, are infrequently served by the classificatory systems devised within the specialist setting. Many health practitioners have no postgraduate training on the psychological and biological management of such difficulties.

This book therefore gives a 'bottom-up', practical overview of mental health. I have distilled psychological, biological and sociological background material and siphoned off anything that is not relevant to primary care. I hope that after the filtration process, the reader will be left with a product that is clearer and more potent than the best of any other home-brew! I aim to demystify the management of common problems and empower the reader to have a more rewarding and fun time at work, and a better ability to cope with the ever-increasing demand and challenge of dealing with multiple physical and mental health issues often brought by a single individual to a time-limited consultation. Some of the content can be used much of the time. I hope, like me, you will find the rest of the material a helpful aide-memoire.

The ideas in this book do not belong to me. I have massaged specialist material to make it more applicable in our setting. Where possible, I have tried to reference original sources of material. I apologise to any who may feel their ideas are being presented as my own.

With the exception of Part Three on psychological tools, there is a logical order to the book. After considering causation, we look at assessment and then take steps down through the various presenting problems as they appear within a 'diagnostic hierarchy'. Where historically there has been a deficit in understanding or training, the relevant chapter will be bulkier. This is also true for problems that are frequently encountered and managed in primary care.

In Part Three on psychological tools I introduce a framework developed from cognitive behaviour therapy, solution-focused and motivational interviewing techniques. Please have fun with this straight away. I hope the positive experience of using the techniques will keep you motivated to continue with the other, more fact-based chapters.

Mark Morris
September 2008

About the author

After graduating in medicine, Mark worked in various medical specialities
with a number of years spent in psychiatry. He became a member of The Royal
College of Psychiatrists and went on to complete the necessary training to
become a general practitioner and achieved membership of The Royal College
of General Practitioners. He feels lucky to be involved in 'whole person' care,
capitalising on longitudinal relationships with patients and knowledge of their
environment while applying both psychological and biological management
strategies. Mark enjoys tailoring specialist skills for application in primary care
and running workshops for primary care practitioners.

Acknowledgements

Thanks to Kate, Elliot and Poppy for their love, patience and fun.

Thank you to the late Dr Dick Ropner, who recognised my perfectionist streak. He insisted that (for me) 'a job worth doing is NOT worth doing properly'!

I am grateful to my parents who encouraged me to make the most of my opportunities and to Inspector Morse who tempered this with 'be careful what you wish for . . . there is always price to pay!'

And to Prem Rawat who showed me the real opportunity that lies within.

I would also like to thank Professor Stephen Rollnick for his insights and allowing the use of Motivational Interviewing; Evan George for his support and agreeing to the inclusion of aspects of The Brief Therapy Practice model in 'Psychological tools – tools for general use'; Dr Vanessa Griffiths for her enthusiasm and material relating to the psychotherapy of addiction; The Royal College of General Practitioners Substance Misuse Unit for content in the drugs and alcohol chapter; Jeff Allison for allowing me to include his 'Reflective Listening: A 5-Minute Review'; Professor Janet Treasure for enabling me to use the salient features of her guide for general practitioners in the eating disorders chapter; Jill Downing for the illustrations; Gillian Nineham for patiently wading through this work and for her helpful editorial guidance.

Background concepts

BIO-PSYCHOSOCIAL BEINGS INTERACTING WITHIN A SYSTEM

Psychological factors and biological factors combine to make us the people we are and determine the illnesses we develop.

Functional (biological) brain scan changes associated with mental disorder are reversed following psychological interventions just as they are after treatment with medications. Research findings relating to cognitive therapy and obsessive-compulsive disorder serve as an example.[1,2] Let us remember that our state of psychological health impacts on us as a whole. Clinical depression thins the bones and increases our risk four-fold of developing diseased coronary arteries.[3] Maternal anxiety is associated with impaired blood flow to the foetus and this may underlie the association between maternal anxiety and small for gestational age babies.[4] These examples show that we no longer have to worry about the philosophical mind-body problem. There is no problem. There are just two different ways of looking at the same thing. We are able to modify the brain with the mind and the mind with the brain; we can influence biology with psychology and psychology with biology. And if we accept that we respond psychologically to our environment (the things we do, where we do them and the people we do them with) we have to also accept that our biology is influenced by our environment. For those who believe the mind is the complex neural circuitry of the brain, there is still the mystery of how social interaction translates into biological change. Accepting that we exist in this rather magical way allows us to have more enjoyable and satisfying collaborations with our patients as we are able to think more holistically about their problems and offer them more choices.

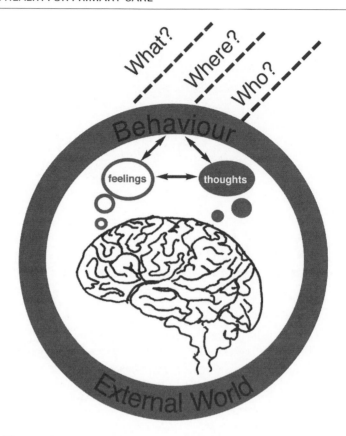

FIGURE A Bio-psychosocial beings

BOX A CASE STUDY

A single mother's recovery from major depression (clinical depression) was largely due to the acquisition of a double buggy! This provided her with the means to take her baby twins to the park where she could engage socially with other parents and their children. Admittedly she needed some low key additional help in the way of a support worker to accompany her to the park the first couple of times. However, in this case, no formal psychological treatment or medication was required. Her persistently and pervasively low mood and symptoms traditionally considered to reflect physiological brain chemistry changes started to shift by being with the 'right people, in the right place, at the right time'. Though medication may have helped to bring about a speedier recovery, it is good to remind ourselves of the other approaches available to help bring about positive change.

VULNERABILITY-STRESS MODEL . . . OR VULNERABILITY/ RESILIENCE STRESS MODEL

The vulnerability-stress model is extremely helpful when considering an individual's mental health issues. Not everybody exposed to stressful circumstances becomes mentally unwell. Illness may occur when stressor(s) interact with personality or biological vulnerability. In the following pages I give consideration to the factors which influence firstly our vulnerability or resilience to illness and then the nature of stressors that can tip us into psychological ill health.

REFERENCES

1. Linden DEJ. How psychotherapy changes the brain – the contribution of functional neuroimaging. *Mol Psychiatry.* 2006; **11**: 528–38.
2. Baxter L, Schwartz JM, Bergman KS, *et al.* Caudate glucose metabolic rate changes with both drug and behaviour therapy for obsessive-compulsive disorder. *Arch Gen Psychiatry.* 1992; **49**: 681–9.
3. Dinan TG. The physical consequences of depressive illness. *BMJ.* 1999; **318**: 826.
4. Teixeira JMA, Fisk NM, Glover V. Association between maternal anxiety in pregnancy and increased uterine artery resistance index: cohort based study. *BMJ.* 1999; **318**: 153–7.

PART ONE

Causation

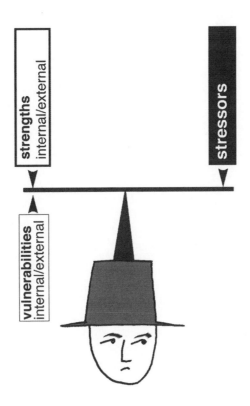

CHAPTER 1

Vulnerability and resilience: personality

We all have vulnerabilities, strengths and resources. These can be external or internal. The fact that I have a relatively high genetic loading for the development of mental illness is an internal vulnerability. However, my training in mental health has made me very aware of this and I should be in a good position to spot the early signs of mental ill health. This is an internal strength. My openness with colleagues and family would help me to access support (external resources). Hopefully, in the face of a stressor the balance of vulnerabilities and strengths will be favourable. If not, neighbours may suffer the sight of me running down the street naked (something my relative did during a manic upswing). The more I think about it, the more important it is for me to bolster my resilience – the mental health of the whole neighbourhood is at stake!

In the field of medicine we often forget to consider the strengths of an individual. In the research, attention is given to weaknesses and vulnerabilities so that we can get a better understanding of the aetiology of mental illness. However, when it comes to moving out of illness or mental distress, strengths and resources are at least as important. Helping individuals to see that they are not the problem and that there is more to them than their difficulties can be very helpful in enabling them to make positive change. It can also be very refreshing for the practitioner.

Let's take a journey from conception through to adulthood, looking at the factors which may have bearing on our mental health.

GENETICS

It would seem that there may be a genetic contribution to all mental illness. Bipolar affective disorder (manic depression) has the greatest heritability.* Family studies show that having a first degree relative with the condition makes you 8–18 times more likely to develop the condition yourself. Adoption studies confirm the genetic contribution by removing confounding environmental factors. To illustrate the point further, the lifetime risk of developing schizophrenia is 1% but having two first degree relatives with schizophrenia increases your risk to 46% (14% with one first degree relative). The genetics are complex and we cannot yet do anything about the loading once it is there. However, in primary care the family make-up is often known to us and we can be alert to genetic vulnerability in the hope of early identification of emerging mental health problems.

Genetics will also have influence over infant temperament as we will discover below.

BIRTH

Obstetric complications and perinatal hypoxia are associated with schizophrenia, particularly in males. Periventricular brain haemorrhages during labour and subsequently enlarged ventricles may be implicated.[2,3]

EARLY RELATIONSHIPS

Figure 1.1 serves as a useful summary – showing that healthy individuals have been provided with safety, security, lots of emotional warmth and a moderate amount of control.

Until the age of three: temperament and attachment
Temperament and 'goodness of fit'

Many early characteristics are inborn. The infant's behaviour can shape parental response, which will in turn influence the child's emotional development. A child who likes cuddling and is easily soothed will promote feelings of competency in the carer and secure attachment will be promoted. The child who stiffens, wriggles and continues to cry when picked up for comfort will make the parent feel inadequate and rejected. There can be negative emotional and behavioural consequences when the child's temperament and family characteristics do not fit nicely together. Thomas and Chess in the 1960s and

---

* Heritability is an estimate of the contribution of genetics to the differences observed in a measured variable (e.g. some dimension of behaviour) in a given population at a given time.

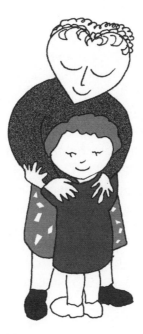

FIGURE 1.1 Early relationships

1970s found that particular characteristics were more likely to remain stable over time than individual characteristics. These clustered together to define the **'difficult child'**[4] – outlined in Table 1.1.

TABLE 1.1 Difficult child

Dimension	Difficult Child Characteristic
Rhythmicity of biological function	No real rhythm (this has been traditionally most bothersome to Mediterranean mums)
Intensity of response	Intense
Prevailing mood	Negative
Approach vs. withdrawal from situations	Withdraw from new situations
Adaptability	Will not adapt

Attachment theory (Bolby,[5] Ainsworth[6])

Attachment theory states that the clinging behaviour which young children display towards their parents is normal and biologically determined, has particular characteristics, and is especially important in psychosocial development. Selective clinging to one person is understood as evidence of an individual's first close personal relationship and it is held that the experience of that relationship will govern the quality of subsequent close relationships throughout life. The quality of attachment will influence future physical and psychological health with an effect on stress regulation mediated by the hypothalamo-pituitary-adrenal axis.[7]

At an average age of about six or seven months, children start to show *attachment behaviours,* which indicate that they are becoming psychologically attached to another person, usually their mother.

The attachment figure is usually someone who has had a lot to do with the baby in terms of play and comforting; feeding is not the crucial element and breast or bottle feeding is simply irrelevant. Even harsh physical treatment or battering is compatible with the development of an attachment to the abuser; it is the intensity of the interaction that matters. Nor is the amount of time spent with a person crucial; what matters is the intensity of social interactions. Working mothers are quite able to elicit attachments from their infants as long as they do things with them at some time during the average day. In practice the first attachment figure is nearly always the baby's mother (or attachment is formed equally with mother and father). After the first attachment, a few other attachments are likely to be formed, particularly to the other parent, but do not have the intensity of the first one.

1 Normal attachment formation

The development of secure affectional bonds in early childhood makes it much more likely that an attitude of trust and optimism in personal relationships will persist in later life.

Normal attachment behaviours compatible with secure attachment formation are identifiable in routine consultations.

In the child normal attachment behaviours comprise:
➤ **separation anxiety**: crying when mother leaves the room; calling for her; crawling or toddling after her. Can interfere with settling at night. Some children find that they can deal with it by having a cuddly toy, known as a comfort object or **transitional object** such as a blanket or teddy bear. Their existence does not indicate insecurity
➤ **clinging** hard when anxious, fearful, tired or in pain, hugging, climbing onto her lap
➤ **talking and playing more in her company**
➤ using her as a **secure base** from which to explore
➤ **stranger anxiety**: wariness towards and shyness of strange people which promotes clinging to the attachment figure in their presence.

Attachment behaviours are intensified by:
➤ **anxiety**
➤ **tiredness**
➤ **illness.**

The mother or carer will be observed *responding sensitively* to the child's needs, providing a sense of security. This promotes adequate resolution of separation anxiety.

Ordinarily speaking, a child gradually learns to tolerate separations so that separation anxiety wanes over the pre-school years, although it will still appear at times of distress and pain in young schoolchildren.

2 *Abnormal attachment formation*
A failure to develop affectional bonds may result in a lack of basic trust with resulting shallowness, suspicion and selfishness in future relationships (and remember this may include the individual's relationship with you!).

It can sometimes be difficult to distinguish between unstable attachment formation and a self-sufficient child. The child may appear very friendly to the examining doctor but closer questioning or longer acquaintance reveals that he or she does not discriminate between familiar and unfamiliar adults in terms of seeking comfort and affection. Although appearing intimate (sitting on your lap, offering kisses), the relationship is superficial and easily broken by separation without any separation anxiety.

The best test is asking the mother if she feels emotionally close to her child
Parental and child factors can lead to abnormal attachment formation. Abnormal attachment patterns have been classified, but I can never remember them. Remembering the following influences may be more useful.

Parental factors
Harshness, coldness or rejection on the part of the parent can promote abnormal attachment behaviour and a poor prognosis for future antisocial behaviour. The situation can be improved if the parent can be persuaded to act in a more sensitive, affectionate and child-centred way, but this is not easy.

When attachment behaviours fail to develop adequately the long-term outcome is often poor with a general difficulty forming and sustaining close relationships, a difficulty learning social rules and a propensity in adult life to aggressive, promiscuous behaviour. These 'immature' adult personality traits fall into the diagnostic categories of psychopathic (antisocial); emotionally unstable ('borderline') personality disorders, and are discussed in Chapter 9.

Child factors

In some instances insecure attachment reflects elements in the child's personality; wriggly children who do not want to hang around on the parental lap for cuddles even though the parents are loving and affectionate. Such a pattern has a good prognosis as long as the parents can accept their child's individuality. There is no strong link with aggressive behaviour.

A bit of both

Children who are chronically clingy and obviously ambivalent to their mother, being actively cross with her following the briefest separations, can result from an unfortunate mix of the child's temperament and mother's state of mind or personality. A depressed and irritable mother, for instance, may be short-tempered with a child and her rejecting attitude promotes further clinging by the child. A mother with an immature personality may find herself unable to separate out her needs from the child's and turn to the child for caring or gratification in a way that makes the child anxious and clingy. Some insecure infants, however, have been exceptionally anxious and irritable throughout their life and have perfectly satisfactory mothers; it is wrong to always blame the child's mother for causing an insecure attachment.

It has generally been held that insecure attachments are likely to precede emotional disorder in childhood, particularly school refusal. Some believe that disorders arising in adolescence or adult life such as agoraphobia also have their roots in insecure attachment formation in early childhood.

The ideal therefore would be for a parent to *consistently respond sensitively to the child's needs while providing a secure base from which the child can explore.* This is most likely to promote secure attachments between the age of six months and three years and a well adjusted adult later on.

As the child continues to grow: style of parenting

Parenting style continues to influence vulnerability by impacting on personality development.

The following poem captures it all:

Children Learn What They Live (1998) by Dorothy Law Nolte (1924–2005)

If children live with criticism, they learn to condemn.
If children live with hostility, they learn to fight.
If children live with fear, they learn to be apprehensive.
If children live with pity, they learn to feel sorry for themselves.

If children live with *ridicule*, they learn to feel shy.
If children live with jealousy, they learn to feel envy.
If children live with *shame*, they learn to feel *guilty*.
If children live with *encouragement*, they learn confidence.
If children live with tolerance, they learn patience.
If children live with *praise*, they learn appreciation.
If children live with acceptance, they learn to love.
If children live with approval, they learn to like themselves.
If children live with recognition, they learn it is good to have a goal.
If children live with sharing, they learn generosity.
If children live with honesty, they learn truthfulness.
If children live with *fairness*, they learn justice.
If children live with *kindness* and consideration, they learn respect.
If children live with security, they learn to have faith in themselves and in those about them.
If children live with friendliness, they learn the world is a nice place in which to live.

> Excerpted from the book *Children Learn What They Live*
> ©1998 by Dorothy Law Nolte and Rachel Harris
> The poem 'Children Learn What They Live'
> ©Dorothy Law Nolte
> Workman Publishing Co., New York.

Behavioural or emotional problems are more likely to emerge where there is:
➤ inconsistent discipline
➤ inconsistent support
➤ anxious overprotection.

Research into 'expressed emotion' has examined the effects of high household levels of:
➤ critical comments (e.g. statements of resentment, disapproval, dislike – reduced emotional warmth)
➤ hostility (criticism for what the person is – reduced emotional warmth)
➤ emotional over-involvement (overprotection, intrusion – i.e. excess control).

The research shows that in these situations an individual may be at increased risk of future depression or relapse into psychotic illness.[8-10] Clearly, such an environment wouldn't help one's self-esteem.

This Expressed Emotion work does seem to complement the following model with its two easy to remember 'style dimensions':
1 **control** dimension
2 **emotional warmth** dimension.

Authoritarian style

High levels of control with low levels of affection yield compliant but withdrawn and dependent children. Self-esteem (evaluation of self-image) is negatively affected. Problems such as depression and disordered eating (from body image, control issues) can emerge from such low self-esteem. Individuals develop with a perception that they lack the capacity to cope with life's demands. This perception causes the stress that can precipitate ill health when facing situations in life. Another way of looking at it is that strict, critical parenting develops a strong superego ('internalised parent'/conscience) with a vulnerability to experiencing guilt and anxiety in later life. This is further explored in the next chapter.

Permissive/laissez-faire style

Low levels of control yield immature children who lack purpose and self-control with an increased risk of future drug or alcohol misuse.

Ideal parenting styles

Emotional well-being is promoted within homes where there is a moderate amount of control and a high score on emotional warmth – an authoritative style of parenting.

This is characterised by the use of parental authority and household rules with some explanation; attending to the child's view; granting some responsibility to the child but retaining veto. Children are more likely to develop independence, assertiveness, creativity and friendliness.[11-13]

Carl Rogers (1902–1987; the founder of client/person centred therapy) introduced the concept of *unconditional positive regard* – people are more likely to become more fully functioning if brought up with unconditional positive regard; they feel themselves valued by parents and others even when their feelings, thoughts (beliefs) and behaviours are less than ideal.[14,15]

Healthy emotional development is also promoted by a *consistent approach* to parenting.

In primary care, longitudinal relationships with families are forged and the practitioner is lucky enough to gain some insight into the interactions that occur with the possibility of shaping patterns for the better.

RESULTANT CORE BELIEFS

The 'cognitive model' (Aaron Beck[16]) hypothesises that people's emotions and behaviours are influenced by their perception of events rather than the situations themselves. Our early experiences such as the quality of early relationships outlined above have bearing on the types of deeply held 'core beliefs' we have about ourselves and the world.

These core beliefs will influence how we respond mentally to situations in life. Negative core beliefs on the left-hand side of the table will lead to worse mental health than the alternative core beliefs opposite them.

TABLE 1.2 Core beliefs

Negative Core Beliefs	Alternative (Healthy) Beliefs
I'm completely unlovable	I'm generally a likeable person
I'm bad	I'm a worthwhile person
I'm powerless	I have control over many things
I'm defective	I'm normal with both strengths and weaknesses

THE USE OF DEFENCE MECHANISMS (ANNA FREUD[17]– DAUGHTER OF SIGMUND)

Defence mechanisms are unconscious strategies that people use to deal with negative emotions. They do not change the stressful situation; they change the way the individual perceives it. We all use them to get us through the rough spots until we can deal more effectively with the stressful situation. *If they become a dominant mode of responding to problems, they can lead to ill health.* The various defence mechanisms are outlined below.

Repression

Impulses and memories that are too frightening or painful are excluded from conscious awareness. Memories that evoke shame, or guilt are often repressed. Feelings that are inconsistent with our self-concept can be repressed e.g. feelings of hostility towards a loved one or feelings of failure.

Suppression is the conscious cousin of repression: keeping impulses and desires in check or temporarily pushing aside painful memories.

We can develop a painful 'emotional abscess' from excessive repression/ suppression of mental events. It has been found that people with a strong repressive/suppressive style have a heightened vulnerability to illness in general including coronary heart disease and more rapid course of cancer. People who confide in others about traumatic events and their associated feelings tend to show better health. There is a recognised rebound effect where suppressed unwanted thoughts come back with greater force when the individual's guard is down. People who suppress more seem to ruminate more often on the distressing thoughts/memories as they return with greater force. In turn, this heightened level of distress and physiological arousal accompanying it could have negative effects on the body.

Rationalisation

Using a good reason rather than a true reason for a course of action. Assigning a socially acceptable or logical motive to what we do to make us feel more comfortable.

Reaction formation

Concealing a motive by giving strong expression to the opposite motive. People who protest with zeal against loose morals or substance misuse may have experienced such problems personally and their current behaviour may be a means of defending themselves against the possibility of slipping backwards into old habits.

Projection

Attributing to others one's own unacceptable or unwanted thoughts or emotions.

Intellectualisation

Dealing with very stressful situations in detached, abstract, intellectual terms. It would become a problem if it generalised into all aspects of life and the individual became emotionally cut off from all emotional experiences.

Displacement/sublimation

A motive that cannot be gratified in one form is directed into a new channel. Hostile impulses may find acceptable expression through contact sport participation.

Denial

When an external reality is too unpleasant to face, an individual may deny that it exists. Sometimes, denying facts may be better than facing them and may give the person time to face the grim facts in a more gradual way, e.g. after sustaining a spinal injury we might give up all together if we were fully aware of the seriousness of the condition. However, denying the presence of say a breast lump may delay presentation to the doctor, leading to a worse prognosis.

Regression

The reversion to an earlier stage of developmental behaviour generally in an attempt to reduce overwhelming anxiety.

BRAIN INSULTS

The term brain insults refers to physical attacks on the brain such as illicit drug use and head injury.

There is a significant statistical association between the smoking of cannabis and the later development of psychotic illness. Though most people who use cannabis do not go on to develop psychosis, there is robust epidemiological evidence supporting a link. This may be particularly relevant to individuals who carry a variant of the catechol-o-methyltransferase (COMT) gene. This gene has a role in regulating brain dopamine concentrations and has been implicated in the development of schizophrenia.[18] This is important information to share with patients.

At the beginning of this chapter we discussed the association between obstetric complications and future psychosis. Research also suggests that non-obstetric related head injury slightly increases the risk of psychosis developing at least 10 years later.[19]

CURRENT RELATIONSHIPS

Protective factors provided by relationships include the following.[20]

A confiding relationship

The presence of a confidant(e) is known to reduce vulnerability to onset and may also protect against recurrence of depression.

Satisfaction with current social network

The characteristics of social support have to be perceived by the individual as adequate, and the support has to be available to them at times of crisis.

REFERENCES

1. McGuffin P, Rijdsdijk F, Andrew M, *et al*. The heritability of bipolar affective disorder and the genetic relationship to unipolar depression. *Arch Gen Psychiatry*. 2003; **60**: 497–502.
2. Hultman CM, Öhman A, Cnattingius S, *et al*. Prenatal and neonatal risk factors for schizophrenia. *Br J Psychiatry*. 1997; **170**: 128–33.

3. Geddes JR, Lawrie SM. Obstetric complications and schizophrenia: a meta-analysis. *Br J Psychiatry*. 1995; **167**: 786–93.
4. Thomas A, Chess S. *Temperament and Development*. New York: Brunner/Mazel; 1977.
5. Bowlby J. *Attachment and Loss*. London: Hogarth Press; 1969.
6. Ainsworth MD, Blehar MC, Waters E, *et al*. *Patterns of Attachment: A Psychological Study of the Strange Situation*. Hillsdale, NJ: Lawrence Erlbaum Associates Inc; 1978.
7. Rees C. Essay – childhood attachment. *Br J Gen Pract*. 2007; **57**(544): 920–2.
8. Bebbington P, Kuipers L. The predictive utility of EE in schizophrenia: an aggregate analysis. *Psychological Medicine*. 1994; **24**: 707–18.
9. Butzlaff RL, Hooley JM. Expressed emotion and psychiatric relapse: a meta-analysis. *Arch Gen Psychiatry*. 1998; **55**: 547–52.
10. Vaughn CE, Leff JP. The influence of family and social factors on the course of psychiatric illness. *Br J Gen Pract*. 1976; **129**: 125–37.
11. Baumrind D. The influence of parenting style on adolescent competence and substance use. *J Early Adolesc*. 1991; **11**(1): 56–95.
12. Weiss LH, Schwarz JC. The relationship between parenting types and older adolescents' personality, academic achievement, adjustment, and substance use. *Child Development*. 1996; **67**(5): 2101–14.
13. Miller NB, Cowan PA, Cowan CP, *et al*. Externalizing in preschoolers and early adolescents: a cross-study replication of a family model. *Developmental Psychology*. 1993; **29**(1): 3–18.
14. Rogers CR. A theory of therapy, personality and interpersonal relationships, as developed in the client-centered framework. In: Koch S, editor. *Psychology: A Study of Science*. New York: McGraw Hill; 1959. pp. 184–256.
15. Rogers CR. *Client-Centred Therapy*. Boston: Houghton Mifflin; 1951.
16. Beck AT. Thinking and depression: II. Theory and therapy. *Arch Gen Psychiatry*. 1964; **10**: 561–71.
17. Freud A. *The Ego and the Mechanisms of Defence*. London: Hogarth Press and Institute of Psycho-Analysis; 1937.
18. Fergusson DM, Poulton R, Smith PF, *et al*. Cannabis and psychosis. *BMJ*. 2006; **332**: 172–5.
19. Harrison G, Whitley E, Rasmussen F, *et al*. Risk of schizophrenia and other non-affective psychosis among individuals exposed to head injury: case control study. *Schizophr Res*. 2006; **88**: 119–26.
20. Alloway R, Bebbington PE. The buffer theory of social support: a review of the literature. *Psychological Medicine*. 1987; **17**: 91–108.

CHAPTER 2

Stressors: precipitating factors

Having considered the variables that influence our vulnerability, we now consider those stressors that can provoke the onset of illness.

NO STRESSORS

Sometimes there are no obvious precipitants to the presenting problem. The term 'endogenous' has been used to mean 'coming from within' when there has been no obvious external stressors triggering the onset of a problem.

EXTERNAL EVENTS

For events to tip the balance we need to perceive them as being stressful, i.e. endangering our physical or psychological well-being. These events tend to be:
➤ uncontrollable
➤ unpredictable
➤ a challenge to one's capabilities and self concept.[1]

This can help us see why our patients and colleagues become stressed or become mentally unwell.

An individual with poorly controlled epilepsy is living with the unpredictability of their fits, not knowing when the next one will be or its consequences. Someone living with a violent alcoholic may feel they have no control over the unpredictable behaviour. The individual may have a self-concept involving self-doubt and feelings of ineffectiveness. Appropriate help might be successful in empowering the individual to take more control over their circumstances by giving them support and options.

The events that drive or complicate the working day of many front-line health professionals are largely uncontrollable and unpredictable.

Lack of control in the workplace can account for a greater percentage of mortalities from all causes than the usual culprits of diet, smoking and exercise. One study found that the lower the employment grade of male civil servants, the higher the incidence of cardiovascular disease. The major factor influencing disease was the level of control the individual had over their work.[2]

There is evidence that after positive or negative life events an individual is more at risk of illness. Moving home can be perceived as positive but the event can be unpredictable.

INTERNAL RESPONSE TO EVENTS

Conditioned response

Pavlov demonstrated 'classical conditioning' by repeatedly pairing the ringing of a bell and the giving of food to his dogs. He was then able to induce salivation in his dogs just by ringing the bell (how lovely!). In a similar way, people may react with fear and anxiety to situations that caused them harm or stress in the past. Many human fears may be acquired in this way, particularly in early childhood and reactivated at some time in the future at a time of stress.[3] The 'primitive' components of the brain known as the amygdala and hippocampus are implicated in the acquisition and maintenance of fear responses.

Cognitive (thinking) style

Thoughts, feelings and behaviours affect each other. We all have different self-concepts and we will appraise events differently. Our thinking styles are rooted in our core beliefs which are formed as a result of early relationships and events (discussed earlier). Extreme negative thoughts will bring about feelings of low mood or anxiety. Our mood states and thinking content will have bearing on our behaviours and activity choices. Different thinking errors are illustrated below.[4]

1 **All-or-nothing thinking (black-and-white thinking)**: thinking of things in absolute terms, like 'always', 'every' or 'never'. Few aspects of human behaviour are so absolute.
2 **Overgeneralisation**: taking isolated cases and using them to make wide generalisations.
3 **Mental filter**: focusing exclusively on certain, usually negative or upsetting, aspects of something while ignoring the rest, like a tiny imperfection in a piece of clothing.

4 **Disqualifying the positive**: continually 'shooting down' positive experiences for arbitrary, ad hoc reasons.

5 **Jumping to conclusions**: assuming something negative where there is no evidence to support it. Two specific subtypes are also identified:

  a   *mind reading* – assuming the intentions of others

  b   *fortune telling* – predicting how things will turn out before they happen.

6 **Magnification** and **minimisation**: inappropriately understating or exaggerating the way people or situations truly are. Often the positive characteristics of *other people* are exaggerated and negative characteristics are understated. There is one subtype of magnification: **catastrophising** – focusing on the worst possible outcome, however unlikely, or thinking that a situation is unbearable or impossible when it is really just uncomfortable.

7 **Emotional reasoning**: making decisions and arguments based on how you *feel* rather than objective reality.

8 **Making 'should' statements**: concentrating on what you think 'should' or ought to be rather than the actual situation you are faced with, or having **rigid rules** which you think should always apply no matter what the circumstances are.

9 **Labelling**: explaining behaviours or events merely by naming them; related to overgeneralisation. Rather than describing the specific behaviour, you assign a label to someone or yourself that puts them in absolute and unalterable terms.

10 **Personalisation**: assuming you or others directly caused things when that may not have been the case. When applied to others this is an example of blame.

When I was training to be a GP it became known that I had an interest in psychological management approaches. I was asked to run a workshop for my peer group. I felt very anxious. I took notice of the thought that had come to mind along with the feeling of anxiety. I established that this 'automatic' thought was 'I cannot do it'. If I had accepted this, I would have behaved in an avoidant way – I would have declined the offer. This would have perpetuated any future anxiety issues in relation to teaching. Instead, I chose to challenge this belief, and identified evidence from past experience that did not fully support my negative thought. This allowed me to form a more balanced view of the situation and with it came a reduction in anxiety and an enjoyable workshop. This methodology is derived from cognitive behaviour therapy and is discussed more thoroughly in the psychological tools chapters.

Mismatch between our behaviours and our beliefs

Cognitive Dissonance Theory states that when an individual engages in behaviour that is counter to their attitudes or beliefs there will be emotional discomfort and a 'dissonance pressure' to change the attitude/belief or the behaviour. (Festinger[5])

Learned helplessness

We see this a lot in people developing depression. Martin Seligman found that animals exposed to repeated stresses that they could not control became understandably a little bit fed up! To be more exact they became passive and behaved like depressed people. This formed the basis of his theory of depression. People who have repeatedly experienced uncontrollable events (yes, the 'control' word again!) may become convinced that nothing they do can control events and they give up.[6]

Instinctive needs or motives in opposition to our developed belief systems

For example, if as a result of negative experiences we have developed a core belief that other people are untrustworthy, there will be conflict with our natural (pack animal) desire for close relationships.

Battling ego

Some of us try harder and are more successful than others at behaving in a culturally acceptable manner and drawing a veil over the fact that we are members of the animal kingdom. It is obvious from the available evidence that a drinking binge puts paid to all that – the shackles provided by our frontal lobes seem cut apart as primitive needs of feeding, fornicating and fighting become very important and these impulses seek gratification with great zeal. The intoxicated often end up on all fours or sleeping in hedges: just further proof of our relationship to other animals!

Sigmund Freud was originally a neurologist. He developed the structural theory of personality which intuitively makes some sense.[7] Essentially, the personality, in his view, consists of three parts:

Id consists of basic biological impulses or drives. These impulses (e.g. the need to eat, drink, gain sexual pleasure, eliminate waste) seek immediate gratification ('The Pleasure Principle').

Superego (nicely represented neurologically by the frontal lobes of the brain) acts as our 'internalised parent'/representation of the values and morals of society; it is our conscience. It judges whether our actions are right or wrong.

Violating the standards of the superego can lead to anxiety or guilt. Individuals who experienced strict, critical parenting (remember parenting styles) are likely to have strong superegos and be more vulnerable to experiencing guilt and anxiety after any minor transgression.

Ego is a buffer and hopefully makes some sensible compromise between these battling factions. It considers the demands of reality and obeys the 'reality principle'. It delays gratification of impulses until the situation is appropriate. It decides which actions are appropriate; which impulses should be satisfied and when.

The defence mechanisms discussed in the previous chapter are used by the ego to reduce conflict between the Id and superego and thereby anxiety. *We are healthy if the Ego remains in firm but flexible control.*

Sex and aggression are two areas in which the Id (impulses) are in conflict with moral standards (superego), causing stress, unless there is too much alcohol on board, in which case the Id wins with no immediate angst to the individual whatsoever!

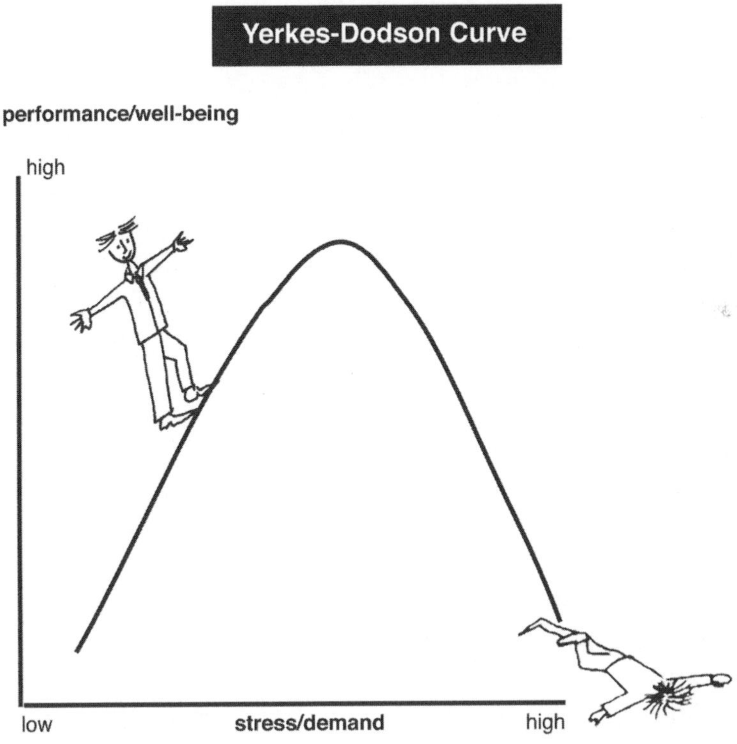

FIGURE 2.1 Yerkes-Dodson Curve

Stress-performance issues

This is particularly useful when discussing causation with patients. It is also usefully applied when we are helping people to pitch demands sensibly during recovery from emotional crises as we will discuss later. The Yerkes-Dodson law predicts an inverted U-shaped function between arousal and performance as shown in Figure 2.1.[8]

Too much or too little challenge will work against us. Research has seen the relevance of the curve to the effects of arousal, anxiety, tension or stress upon learning, performance, problem solving, coping or memory. I know that I thrive with a certain amount of challenge (demand/stress); my self-esteem is bolstered as I perform well. As someone who likes a job done properly, as the demand is increased beyond a critical point, I end up trying to do too much, too well and in too short a space of time. This becomes impossible, my performance slips and I risk becoming tense and irritable.

BIOLOGY

The hypothalamic-pituitary-adrenal system

So what are the biological events that are paired with these psychological phenomena?

When we are stressed, the brain sends hormonal and neuronal (sympathetic nervous system) messages to the adrenal glands (sitting on top of the kidneys). These result in the release of the stress hormones adrenalin and cortisol.

In an acutely stressful situation involving a serious immediate threat it is natural to experience the effects of adrenalin on our bodies. The heart tends to go like the clappers; we sweat and start to breathe more rapidly and blood is diverted to our muscles. All of this is useful if we have to run for our lives from a predator. The problem for us arises if this response happens when there is no serious threat. Having trouble getting air into your lungs, sweating like a pig, feeling light headed, having a dry mouth, trouble swallowing, wobbly legs and wobbly voice are a real inconvenience and often very distressing if they occur inappropriately as they do in a panic disorder (occurs out of the blue – unrelated to specific situations). It can also be unhelpful when it happens in specific situations that have become a threat that really shouldn't be (when there is a specific phobic anxiety).

Cortisol is released as a response to the adrenocorticotrophic hormone (ACTH) that is sent from the pituitary gland in the brain. The pituitary gland does this because the hypothalamus in the brain tells it to by sending corticotrophic releasing hormone (CRH) when we are stressed. Cortisol is helpful in many ways: it mobilises energy reserves when we need them and works as an anti-inflammatory agent. Its dampening down of many immune functions such as reducing the number of macrophages and monocytes (part of the circulating surveillance system), inhibiting cytokine production and blocking inflammatory mediators is without risk in the short term. Under normal conditions the release of cortisol is tightly regulated by negative feedback mechanisms that monitor levels in the body and act to shut down production at an appropriate time. So, when a stress has passed or an immune challenge (such as a bacterial invasion) negated, balance is restored.

The lower grade workers with less control over their work environment that were discussed earlier expressed lower work satisfaction and more chronic strain. This chronic stress was reflected in major physiological changes such as elevated cortisol levels (reflecting hypothalamic-pituitary-adrenal (HPA) axis activation) and increased blood lipid levels (cholesterol and triglycerides). This in turn led to an increased incidence of cardiovascular disease, diabetes and depression. Cortisol modulates the transmission of our brain mood chemicals (dopamine, noradrenalin and most particularly serotonin). It has been shown that many depressed people have an HPA system stuck in high gear. After an episode of major depression the risk of developing coronary heart disease is increased four-fold![9] The response to stress also increases sympathetic nervous system activity. Heart rate and blood pressure are elevated to increase blood supply and energy to the muscles. However, the increase in blood pressure increases wear and tear on blood vessels, providing sites for disease processes to begin. Fat, glucose and foam cells work their way under the lining layer and stick to form plaques resulting in atherosclerosis. Anxiety and post traumatic stress disorder are also linked to activation of the HPA axis. Unfortunately, confronting daily stress and hassle in the 21st century does not provide an opportunity for the energy mobilised by the cortisol to be used. Instead, energy is released from stores into the blood stream and then stored again. This is not only very inefficient, but it also has potential consequences for health. The increase in glucose concentrations in the blood can result in insulin resistance and an increased risk of type II diabetes.[10-14]

Brain insults

Again, drugs come to mind (literally!).

Taking stimulant drugs such as amphetamines, cocaine and methylene-dioxymethamphetamine (MDMA or ecstasy) can cause anxiety, depression, confusional states and paranoid psychotic symptoms.[15]

Cannabis is available with greater concentrations of tetrahydrocannabinol (THC) and it is becoming increasingly common for individuals to develop an enduring psychosis following just a single cannabis indulgence. Cannabis intoxication can lead to acute transient psychotic episodes[16] and cannabis use increases the risk of relapse in people with schizophrenia.[17] There is now more evidence of the association between cannabis use and onset of psychotic disorders.[18]

BEING MENTALLY HEALTHY: A SUMMARY

We are more likely to be mentally healthy if we:
➤ have helpful genes
➤ have an easy birth
➤ have a temperament that fits nicely into our early environment
➤ have parents who consistently respond sensitively to our needs
➤ have parents who provide a secure base from which to explore
➤ have parents who exert a moderate amount of control and at the same time provide lots of emotional warmth
➤ have parents who provide unconditional positive regard
➤ have parents who provide a consistent approach
➤ avoid 'brain insults', e.g. illicit drugs
➤ have satisfying social networks
➤ have confiding relationship(s)
➤ develop healthy core beliefs as a result of the above
➤ do not overuse defence mechanisms
➤ stay clear of environments that throw at us lots of events that we perceive as being
  – out of our control
  – unpredictable
  – a challenge to our capabilities and self-concept
➤ maintain a balanced view of events and our circumstances
➤ manage any mismatch between our behaviours/instinctive needs/ environment and our beliefs
➤ have an ego that remains in firm but flexible control.

REFERENCES

1. Lazarus RS, Folkman S. *Stress, Appraisal, and Coping.* New York: Springer; 1984.
2. Jacobs WJ, Nadel W. Stress-induced recovery of fears and phobias. *Psychological Review.* 1985; **92**: 512–31.
3. Bosma H, Marmot MG, Hemingway H, *et al.* Low job control and risk of coronary heart disease in the Whitehall II (prospective cohort) study. *BMJ.* 1997; **314**: 558–65.
4. Beck AT. *Cognitive Therapy and the Emotional Disorders.* International Universities Press Inc; 1975.

5. Festinger L. *A Theory of Cognitive Dissonance.* Stanford University Press; 1957.
6. Seligman MEP. *Helplessness: On Depression, Development, and Death.* San Francisco: WH, Freeman; 1975.
7. Freud S. *The Ego and the Id.* London: The Hogarth Press Ltd; 1949.
8. Yerkes RM, Dodson JD. The relation of strength of stimulus to rapidity of habit-formation. *Journal of Comparative Neurology and Psychology.* 1908; **18**: 459–82.
9. Dinan TG. The physical consequences of depressive illness. *BMJ.* 1999; **318**: 826–826.
10. Brunner EJ, Hemingway H, Walker BR, *et al.* Adrenocortical, autonomic, and inflammatory causes of the metabolic syndrome-nested case-control study. *Circulation.* 2002; **106**: 2659–65.
11. Steptoe A, Brunner E, Marmot M. Stress-induced inflammatory responses and risk of the metabolic syndrome: a longitudinal analysis. *Obes Res.* 2004; **12**: A76.
12. Bjorntorp P. Visceral fat accumulation – the missing link between psychosocial factors and cardiovascular disease. *J Intern Med.* 1991; **230**: 195–201.
13. Phillips DIW, Barker DJP, Fall CHD, *et al.* Elevated plasma cortisol concentrations: a link between low birth weight and the insulin resistance syndrome? *J Clin Endocrinol Metab.* 1998; **83**: 757–60.
14. Chandola T, Brunner E, Marmot M. Chronic stress at work and the metabolic syndrome: prospective study. *BMJ.* 2006; **332**: 521–4.
15. Seivewright N, McMahon C, Egleston P. Stimulant use still going strong. Revisiting: misuse of amphetamines and related drugs. *Advances in Psychiatric Treatment.* 2005; **11**: 262–9.
16. D'Souza C, Cho HS, Perry E, *et al.* A cannabinoid model psychosis, dopamine-cannabinoid interactions and implications for schizophrenia. In: Castle DJ, Murray R, editors. *Marijuana and Madness.* Cambridge: Cambridge University Press; 2004. pp. 142–65.
17. Treffert D. Marijuana use in schizophrenia: a clear hazard. *Am J Psychiatry.* 1978; **135**: 1213–15.
18. Arseneault L, Cannon M, Witton J, *et al.* Causal association between cannabis and psychosis: examination of the evidence. *Br J Psychiatry.* 2004; **184**: 110–7.

PART TWO

Problems

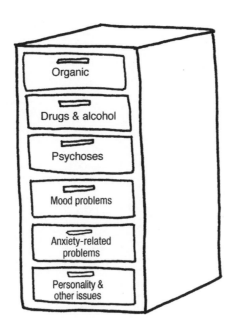

Organic

Drugs & alcohol

Psychoses

Mood problems

Anxiety-related problems

Personality & other issues

CHAPTER 3

Assessment

The aim of assessment is to establish why this particular problem is showing itself in this person at this time. Even though time is often short in primary care there is the opportunity for more frequent encounters than that available for the specialist. It is also often the case that the professional already benefits from some understanding of past and present social issues, which makes assessment easier.

DIAGNOSTIC HIERARCHY

> 'A neurotic builds a castle in the sky; a psychotic lives in it and the psychiatrist calls for the rent.'

This old saying introduces us to the concept of a diagnostic hierarchy. The term 'neurotic' was used to mean any condition in which anxiety or emotional problems were prominent and is no longer considered useful. Someone suffering from psychosis is really losing touch with reality. A psychiatrist is a psychiatrist!

The use of a hierarchy is helpful when we are trying to define the type of presenting problem. In the hierarchy, organic problems (problems where there are obvious structural/physical causes) are at the top and personality issues are at the bottom. Any problem can include features of any of the problems below it in the hierarchy. During an assessment, it is worth considering all the diagnostic possibilities from the top down. For example, a person presenting with pervasive low mood, loss of energy and motivation may have a thyroid problem (an organic problem) rather than primary depressive illness. A disinhibited person with grandiose delusions may have a frontal lobe brain tumour causing the symptoms and signs of mania rather than a mood disorder. Once you have identified the correct hierarchical level for the problem you can enquire about symptoms from the levels below.

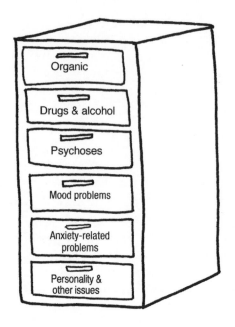

FIGURE 3.1 Diagnostic hierarchy

ONION CONCEPT

The diagnostic hierarchy is complemented by my 'onion concept'. The core of the onion represents the personality. It is hard, deeply ingrained and less easily changed. It may provide a predisposition to illness. The outer onion layers, representing mental illness, are more easily peeled away. Stress and illness can exacerbate the individual's pre-morbid personality characteristics. For example, patients with dramatic, emotionally unstable personality traits often become more histrionic and impulsive during a depressive illness. Removing the depressive illness layer will leave us with someone who is still prone to low self-esteem and emotional instability. These personality characteristics will take longer to change.

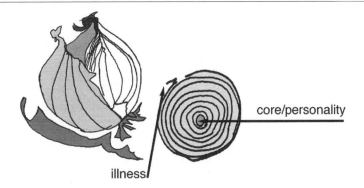

FIGURE 3.2 'Onion concept'

CONSULTATION STYLE AND STRUCTURE
Considering the presenting problem
Keeping quiet and listening
Giving the person uninterrupted time to give their story and reason for attendance aids rapport building and the gathering of accurate information. Research on the detection of depression shows that practitioners who give eye contact, less interruption and appear to be less hurried (i.e. good actors!) are best at the job.

'Scissors questioning'
Start with questions that are likely to receive a long answer, that require the patient to reflect and also hand control of the conversation to the patient. These are *open questions* and they often begin with *'why'*, *'how'*, or *'what'*.

> 'How can I help today?'
> 'How have you been feeling lately?'
> 'How did it all start?'
> 'What was it like?'
> 'What else would you like to mention?'

Next, close down with questions that can be answered with either a single word or a short phrase in order to test your diagnostic ideas – *closed questions*.

> 'Are you able to enjoy things as much as you used to?'

> 'Are you as interested in gardening as you were? Do you enjoy it as much? How long has it been like this?'

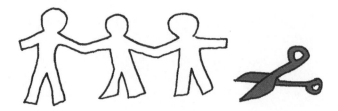

FIGURE 3.3 Scissors questioning

After opening and closing the scissors enough to have gained a good insight into the current symptom pattern we can use further closed questioning to carry out a review: finding out about other physical and psychological and social factors and enquiring about any symptoms from the other levels of the diagnostic hierarchy. Useful direct questions along with other information and advice are provided in subsequent chapters.

Suicide risk

Whatever the hierarchical level, it is always important to address the issue of suicidality.

> 'How do you see the future?'
> 'Has life seemed quite hopeless?'
> 'Can you see any future?'
> 'Have you given up or does there still seem some reason for trying?'
> 'Have you felt that life wasn't worth living?'
> 'Did you ever feel like ending it all?'
> 'What did you think you might do?'
> 'Did you actually try?'

Distress, dysfunction and risk

Find out how the problem is affecting them and other people. Find out if the problem poses a risk to the health and safety of the individual or poses any risk to the safety of others. Risk may be related to the *nature* of the problem or the *degree/severity* of the problem.

Family, personal and social history

The following are useful points to cover.
➤ Family history of mental health problems.
➤ The family structure.

➤ Parenting – *'Did you receive good care from your parents?'* This question is a non-threatening way of beginning a conversation about upbringing, parenting style, attachment issues etc.
➤ Schooling.
➤ Friends in childhood and whether the patient felt part of the peer group.
➤ Academic achievement.
➤ Further education.
➤ Employment history.
➤ Forensic history – *'Have you ever been in trouble with the police?'* Note past offences and terms of prison sentences.
➤ The presence or absence of social supports.
➤ Level of satisfaction with current social circumstances (a lack of satisfaction and social isolation is associated with depression).
➤ The presence or absence of confiding relationships (absence associated with depression).

Premorbid personality

Here we are considering the deeply ingrained features of the individual's character. This has bearing on how the person relates to the world and is influenced by the factors covered in Chapter 1. The presenting problem may simply be an exacerbation of existing personality traits brought about by stress or otherwise a mental condition predisposed to by personality.

The following areas can be considered.

1 Relationships – ability to form and sustain close relationships.
2 Moods/Affect – any tendency to low mood/any evidence of affective instability. *Affect* means immediate 'mood' whereas *mood* refers to the prevailing state. Affective instability refers to the situation where someone can experience sudden changes in their feelings. People with emotionally unstable/'borderline' personalities can go from feeling quite happy one minute to suddenly feeling low, tense with feelings of self-hate and anger.
3 Response to stress.
4 Interests and hobbies – there may be a preference for group activities or for solitary activities.

Drugs and alcohol

Ask about past and present use of alcohol, tobacco and illicit drugs. Explore the route of administration; for example, whether a drug has been smoked or injected. For more details, *see* Chapter 5.

Medical history

Medical problems do not only directly cause mental symptoms e.g. hypothyroidism causes low mood; hyperthyroidism causes agitation and anxiety; Parkinson's disease causes depressed mood through depletion of dopaminergic transmission and the restriction on lifestyle caused by the illness. In Chapter 2 we discussed how events perceived as being unpredictable and out of our control are most likely to precipitate ill health and a number of physical illnesses can have unpredictable effects.

Medications

Many medications have effects on mental state.

Mental state examination

Here we need to consider the following areas that are given more detailed coverage in the following pages.

Appearance and behaviour – areas to consider

Clothing, the amount of eye contact, body movements, whether behaviour seems appropriate to the situation, how easy it is to establish rapport; visible signs of systemic illness.

Speech

Rate and volume.

Thought

Content (preoccupations; obsessions; delusions); form (is it coherent; can you understand what is being said?).

Mood/affect

Does the patient's immediate mood state react during the interview, i.e. is there a change in facial expression, tone of voice and body language in response to changing content of discussion? Somebody with significant depressive illness may not show any change. They might continue to give poor eye contact, give short answers and remain monotonal despite coverage of material that most people consider to be light-hearted.

Is the mood congruent (appropriate to the content of the discussion)? In schizophrenia the immediate mood state might be quite inappropriate.

Perception

Does the patient seem distracted by anything that you cannot see or hear? A distracted patient may be hallucinating.

Insight

How does the patient explain what is going on? Do they think they have a mental health problem?

'ICE' – ideas, concerns and expectations

This is a useful addition to the traditional mental state examination. It is important to ask the patient what they think is happening, what their concerns are and what they think should or shouldn't be done.

Some examples of mental state examination findings

Unremarkable

'At interview, Mr Healthy was clean and casually dressed. He maintained good eye contact and rapport was easily established. Speech was spontaneous and normal in rate and volume. He gave appropriate answers of good length. Thoughts were normal in form and content with no evidence of obsessions or delusions. No evidence of passivity or control phenomena. His affect was reactive during the interview and congruent. There was no evidence of perceptual disturbance and he denied experiencing anything untoward. He did not consider anything to be wrong with his mental health . . . I later realised I had been interviewing the wrong person!'

Depression?

'At interview, Eeyore (remember the donkey from *Winnie-the-Pooh* – always down in the dumps) was unshaven and looked dishevelled. His coat was dirt-stained. He seemed uncomfortable and initially nervous, making it clear that he felt he was wasting my time. However, after reassurance he calmed and rapport was easily established. Eye contact was poor. He lacked facial expression. Speech lacked spontaneity. His answers were short, quiet and monotonal but appropriate to the questions asked. Form of thought was normal. It was difficult to gain access to the content of his thoughts as he said so little; however, on further questioning he revealed a preoccupation with having no role in the Hundred-Acre Wood and believed he was a useless and ineffective donkey. He blamed himself for Tigger losing his bounce despite evidence that Tigger's tail had been cut off in a car accident which had not involved Eeyore in any way. He was ambivalent about life, saying that it was only because of being a coward that he had not ended his life. He was not actively suicidal. He admitted to feeling low; mood was congruent. He did not appear distracted but on further questioning he described hearing a derogatory voice outside of his head directing nasty comments at him. Eeyore considered himself to be depressed and would accept help but was concerned about being prescribed antidepressants because Owl told him they were addictive.'

Summarise

Feeding back the salient features of the problem gives the patient the chance to check that you have heard them correctly and have an accurate description.

Share provisional formulation ideas

Consider together why this particular problem is showing itself at this time. Think about the predisposing, precipitating and perpetuating factors covered in Part One of this book. These factors may be biological, psychological or social. A 'formulation table' might assist you with this exercise. Table 3.1 is a formulation table containing information that might have been relevant to a presentation of depression. It is not always possible to complete all the sections of the table.

TABLE 3.1 Formulation table

	Psychological	Biological	Social
Predisposing	Low self-esteem, self-criticism (understandable given emotionally distant, strict parenting)	e.g. genetic loading – family history of depression	
Precipitating		Possible hypothyroidism	Near death of friend Work issues; loss of control
Maintaining	Extreme negative self-appraisal particularly relating to achievement at work	Has started drinking above the recommended amount of alcohol	Ongoing work problems Social isolation

Example of traditional case formulation

'Eeyore is suffering from major depression (clinical depression) as defined by the DSM-IV criteria. He is predisposed to this by genetic loading (two first degree relatives with major depressive illness), premorbid personality characterised by low self-esteem, a tendency to self-doubt, and self-criticism, which is understandable given the emotionally distant, strict parenting he received as a young donkey. This episode has been precipitated by the near death of his friend Tigger and increasing demands in the workplace where Eeyore has felt an increasing loss of control over an escalating amount of work. He has some symptoms of hypothyroidism which could be contributing to his depressed state. The work issues continue and are maintaining his low mood as is the social isolation that has resulted from his depression.'

What this traditional formulation does not highlight are the resources and strengths that Eeyore has utilised during his life. Although quiet, he has been sociable and has valued friendships. He has cultivated a social support system within the Hundred-Acre Wood which could be usefully utilised during recovery. He has a willpower that got him through past traumas. This combined with his dry sense of humour may help him through this depression. The psychological tools chapters help us to uncover these strengths and resources.

Remember that long-term issues can be exacerbated by illness. For example, in a clinical depression, suppressed thoughts and feelings concerning past trauma/abuse can come to the fore and cause considerable distress. With treatment of the depression, these mental experiences often melt into the background again.

Deciding whether to address past traumas can wait until the depressive illness layer has been peeled away. Addressing such predisposing issues could form an intermediate/long-term part of the management plan. If the patient finds themselves functioning happily again, they may not wish to tackle their vulnerability by opening such a can of worms – once the lid is off, it is hard to shut the contents away again. It can be overwhelming and very distressing. We should not assume that it is for everyone to 'dig and delve'.

Agreed plan of action

Try to agree on a plan of action.

With the patient's consent, obtaining collateral history from a relative or friend can be very useful. Remember that the patient's mental state may well be clouding their view of events and current circumstances.

Consider physical investigations and examination.

Table 3.2 is an example of a 'management plan table'.

TABLE 3.2 Management plan

	Psychosocial	Biological
Short-term management	For example:	For example:
	For milder depression favour psychological treatments such as cognitive behaviour therapy over biological (medication) in the short term.	For more severe depression antidepressant medication would be justified in the short term.
	Brief anxiety management strategies to cope with panic attacks.	Jogging with friend.
	Learning mindfulness meditation to give the patient a sense of distance from their problem thoughts and feelings, and better control over them.	Treat any contributing physical illness.
	Application for a change of housing.	
	Activity scheduling – graded activity.	
	Accessing suitable social support – support group; attending evening art class at local college.	
Intermediate/ longer term management	For example:	For example:
	Work on any significant predisposing factors such as thinking styles/ attachment issues.	Consider maintenance antidepressant treatment for recurrent severe depression.

CHAPTER 4

Dementia and delirium/acute confusional state

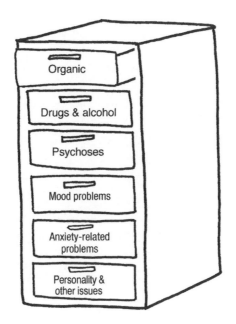

DEMENTIA

Dementia is a set of symptoms: There is evidence of a decline in memory and thinking which is of a degree sufficient to impair functioning in daily living, present for six months or more. This may be accompanied by a decline in emotional control, social behaviour, motivation and/or higher cortical functions.

The onset of dementia may be from age 45, but usually not before 65.

With the growing tendency for people to live longer, it is becoming more important for us to have skills in the assessment and management of dementia.

Assessment

Questions for the patient and carer/relative:

> 'Have you noticed any change in personality?'
> 'Have you noticed any increased forgetfulness?'
> 'Have any activities been given up? Why?'
> 'Has there been any confusion or muddling at night?'
> 'Have there been any problems recognising people?'
> 'Have there been any difficulties with speech?'
> 'Have the changes been gradual or has there been sudden worsening?'

Screening tools

Mini mental state examination[1] – see Appendix 3

This is a screening test for dementia. The patient's verbal fluency, age, education, and social group can all influence the test score. The test takes only about 10 minutes, but is limited because it will not detect subtle memory losses, particularly in well educated patients.[2] People from different cultural groups or low intelligence or education may score poorly on this examination in the absence of cognitive impairment[3] and well educated people may score well despite having cognitive impairment.[4]

➤ Scores of >26 make a diagnosis of dementia unlikely.
➤ Scores of 21–26 may indicate mild dementia.
➤ Scores of 10–20 may indicate moderate dementia.
➤ Scores of <10 usually indicate severe dementia.

When a cut-off of 24 points is used, the mini mental state examination has a sensitivity of 87% and a specificity of 82% in white populations.

Clock drawing test

The patient is asked to draw a clock and then write in the numbers 1–12.

An inability to complete the test has a diagnostic sensitivity of 87% and specificity of 93% for Alzheimer's disease. If the patient's ability to draw the hands of the clock at 11:20 is included, the sensitivity and specificity are increased further.[5]

Remember the hierarchy

Particularly as the dementia progresses, psychiatric symptoms may develop that take on a variety of characteristics resembling discrete mental disorders such as psychosis, mania, depression or anxiety. However, the course and features are more difficult to predict, and treatments are less reliably effective than when these disorders occur in younger adults without dementia. Depressive symptoms are common and often manifest as apathy or a lack of interest in previously enjoyable activities. This depressive syndrome may also include a loss of interest in self-care, eating, or interacting with peers. A propensity for irritability and impulsivity may also occur.

Remember to examine and investigate for delirium (acute confusional state) if there is a rapid onset or fluctuating cognitive impairment.

Dementia threshold

A brain may be affected by any number of pathologies. Once the level of assault reaches a certain threshold, dementing signs may appear. The commonest types of dementia are considered to be Alzheimer's disease, Lewy body disease (a sort of cortical Parkinson's disease) and vascular dementia. However, there may be overlap with an individual suffering vascular damage along with the changes of Alzheimer's disease. The 'E4' gene found on chromosome 14 increases the risk of Alzheimer's disease by coding for the apolipoprotein E contained in the 'plaques and tangles' of an Alzheimer's diseased brain. The same gene also increases the risk of a vascular component to dementia through increasing the cholesterol level.

In the majority of Lewy body brains there are the 'plaques and tangles' associated with Alzheimer's disease. Lewy body disease might actually be a spectrum disorder related to both Alzheimer's and Parkinson's disease – there are cortical Lewy bodies in most Parkinson's diseased brains.

Alzheimer's disease

There tends to be a gradual non step-wise decline.

Anticholinesterase medication may help.[6] These medications boost the transmission of acetylcholine in the brain. A reduction in the quantity of brain cells that are involved in the release of acetylcholine has been associated with Alzheimer's disease.[7] A typical improvement seen from these 'cognitive enhancers' is a 1–2 point rise in the score on the mini mental state examination over a period of six months; this compares with an average decline of 5–6 points over six months in patients who do not take such drugs.[8] However, it is the improvement in social functioning and quality of life that seems more important and has been most noticeable to families and carers. Early referral to a specialist team is important in dementia to establish whether prescription of these medications is appropriate.

Vascular dementia

There are likely to be cardiovascular risk factors (diabetes, hypertension, smoking, raised blood cholesterol/triglycerides).

There is likely to be a 'step-wise decline'.

There may be emotional lability especially at night.

Antiplatelet therapy and tackling cardiovascular risk factors may prevent further decline.

Lewy body disease

There is often a fluctuating course. Other features include visual hallucinations and parkinsonism symptoms and signs.

Antipsychotics may be contraindicated due to bringing on marked extra-pyramidal side-effects in these patients.

Blood investigations for rare causes or complicating conditions

Urea and electrolytes, glucose, lipids, blood count, liver function tests (including GGT), thyroid function, C-reactive protein, vitamin B12, folic acid, syphilis serology.

Rare reversible causes of dementia

These include:

➤ thyroid disease
➤ parathyroid disease
➤ normal pressure hydrocephalus
➤ syphilis
➤ brain tumour
➤ renal failure.
➤ vitamin B12/folic acid deficiency
➤ severe anaemia
➤ anticonvulsant toxicity.

Early referral

If dementia is suspected, early referral to the specialist services is important. Not only does this allow identification of the supportive and social care needs of both carer and patient, but it will also prompt assessment for the suitability of medications – the acetylcholinesterase inhibitors as discussed above.

Non-pharmacological approaches to dementia care

We can encourage employment of the following by carers and nursing/residential home establishments.

Behavioural therapy

A patient with dementia may exhibit problematic behaviours such as physical aggression, wandering, verbal outbursts, resistance to bathing or other care needs, and restless motor activity such as pacing or rocking.

These behaviours may be secondary to other conditions in the hierarchy as outlined above and treatments can be directed at these specific problems. Sometimes, however, the behaviour is due to the dementia. It is important to attempt identification of antecedents, behaviours and consequences (ABC). It can be helpful to suggest the use of a diary or chart to gather information about the manifestations of behaviour and the sequence of actions leading up to it. Environmental triggers might include disruptions in routine, time change (e.g. with daylight savings time or travel across time zones), changes in the care giving environment, new carers, a life stressor (e.g. death of a spouse or family member), over-stimulation (e.g. too much noise, crowded rooms, close contact with too many people), under-stimulation (e.g. relative absence of people, spending much time alone, use of television as a companion), and the disruptive behaviour of other patients. To modify the behaviour we can aim to change the context in which the behaviour takes place and use reinforcement strategies and schedules that reduce the behaviour. The efficacy of formalised behavioural therapy has been demonstrated in the context of dementia in only a small number of studies.[9]

Remember, for our elderly patients the antecedents or triggers may be internal as well as external. Here I am thinking that a physical change such as constipation, pain, infection and medication side-effects can alter behaviour.

Reality orientation

This aims to help people with memory loss and disorientation by reminding them of facts about themselves and their environment. It can be used both with individuals and with groups. In either case, people with memory loss are oriented to their environment using a range of materials and activities. This involves consistent use of orientation devices such as signposts, notices and other memory aids. This approach has been favourably reviewed[10] though there have been some background concerns about the potential impact on self-esteem and mood of reminding people of their deterioration.

Reminiscence therapy

Reminiscence therapy involves helping a person with dementia to relive past experiences, especially those that might be positive and personally significant; for example, family holidays and weddings. This therapy can be used with groups or with individuals. Group sessions tend to use activities such as art, music and artefacts to provide stimulation. This approach may not improve cognitive measures[11] but there may be improvements in behaviour, well-being, social interaction, self-care and motivation.[12]

Music therapy

Several studies have reported benefits gained by people with dementia from music therapy involving engagement in a musical activity (e.g. singing or playing an instrument), or merely listening to songs or music.[13] People with dementia who are played an individualised programme of music as opposed to traditional relaxation music are more likely to experience reduced agitation.[14]

Exercise

Daytime exercise has been shown to help reduce daytime agitation and night-time restlessness.[15]

Aromatherapy

The two main essential oils used in aromatherapy for dementia are extracted from lavender and Melissa balm. There are several routes of administration such as inhalation, bathing, massage and topical application in a cream. This means that the therapy can be targeted at individuals with different behaviours: inhalation may be more effective than massage for a person with restlessness, for instance. There have been some positive results from recent controlled trials which have shown significant reductions in agitation, with excellent compliance and tolerability.[16]

The psychological effects of aromatherapy relate to the individual's perception of the pleasantness of an odour and their past association with an odour. Neurochemical effects have been linked to inhibition of glutamate binding, GABA augmentation and acetylcholine receptor binding.[17]

Pharmacological approaches to dementia care

Medications should only be used to control behaviour as a first line if there is severe distress or risk of harm to the patient or others. In all other cases an assessment of ABC should take place as outlined above and behavioural management strategies should be employed.

Antipsychotics

There is a possible increased risk of cerebrovascular adverse events with the use of antipsychotics and they should not be used for mild-moderate disturbance. In 2004, the UK Committee on Safety of Medicines advised that 'risperidone and olanzapine should not be used for the treatment of behavioural symptoms of dementia'. The decision was based on a summary of clinical data on cerebrovascular adverse events from four randomised controlled trials of risperidone (0.5–2 mg daily) involving a total of 1779 patients with dementia. Patients with Lewy body dementia are at increased risk of extrapyramidal side-effects (*see* Chapter 5) from antipsychotics. Antipsychotic medications may accelerate cognitive decline.[18]

Benzodiazepines

There is some limited evidence that benzodiazepines can help with restlessness and agitation but research has only really focused on the short-term effect of intramuscular lorazepam for severe disturbance rather than longer term oral medication. Of course there are a number of potential negative effects including sedation, worsening memory, dizziness and dependency.[19,20]

Baseline cognitive measures should be taken along with documentation of the severity of problem symptoms before medication treatment starts. There should be early review after starting medication to assess any side-effects. Review of cognitive function and effectiveness of medication at alleviating the target problems should take place regularly (at least every three months). The dose should be low initially and then titrated upwards.

DELIRIUM/ACUTE CONFUSION STATE

A clouding of consciousness (reduced awareness of surroundings) with abrupt onset and markedly fluctuating course.

There is usually an abrupt onset. There is often a fluctuating confusion. The patient might be distressed. Visual hallucinations are often present.

The assessment should be directed at eliciting the cause. The commonest causes are:

➤ urinary tract infections
➤ chest infections
➤ infections of the skin or ear
➤ cardiac failure
➤ medications.

REFERENCES

1. Folstein MF, Folstein SE, McHugh PR. 'Mini-mental state'. A practical method for grading the cognitive state of patients for the clinician. *J Psychiatr Res.* 1975; **12**(3): 189–98.
2. Small GW. What we need to know about age related memory loss. *BMJ.* 2002; **324**(7352): 1502–5.

3. Tombaugh TN, McIntyre NJ. The mini-mental state examination: a comprehensive review. *J Am Geriatr Soc.* 1992; **40**(9): 922–35.
4. Brayne C, Calloway P. The association of education and socioeconomic status with the Mini Mental State Examination and the clinical diagnosis of dementia in elderly people. *Age Ageing.* 1990; **19**(2): 91–6.
5. Wolf-Klein G, Silverstone F, Levy A, *et al.* Screening for Alzheimer's disease by clock drawing. *J Am Geriatr Soc.* 1989; **37**: 730–6.
6. Kelly CA, Harvey RJ, Cayton H. Drug treatments for Alzheimer's disease. *BMJ.* 1997; **314**: 693–4.
7. Bartus RT, Dean RL, Beer B, *et al.* The cholinergic hypothesis of geriatric memory dysfunction. *Science.* 1982; **217**: 408–14.
8. Lyketsos C, Lee H. Diagnosis and treatment of depression in Alzheimer's disease: a practical update for the clinician. *Dement Geriatr Cogn Disord.* 2004; **17**: 55–64.
9. Burgio L, Fisher S. Application of psychosocial interventions for treating behavioural and psychological symptoms of dementia. *Int Psychogeriatr.* 2000; **12**: 351–8.
10. Spector A, Orrell M, Davies S, *et al.* Reality orientation for dementia. *Cochrane Library,* Issue 3. Oxford: Update Software; 2002.
11. Spector A, Orrell M, Davies S, *et al.* Reminiscence therapy for dementia. *Cochrane Library,* Issue 3. Oxford: Update Software; 2002.
12. O'Donovan S. The memory lingers on. *Elder Care.* 1993; **5**: 27–31.
13. Killick J, Allan K. The arts in dementia care: tapping a rich resource. *Journal of Dementia Care.* 1999; **7**: 35–8.
14. Gerdner L. Effects of individualized versus classical 'relaxation' music on the frequency of agitation in elderly persons with Alzheimer's disease and related disorders. *Int Psychogeriatr.* 2000; **12**: 49–65.
15. Alessi C, Yoon E, Schnelle J, *et al.* A randomised trial of a combined physical activity and environment intervention in nursing home residents: do sleep and agitation improve? *J Am Ger Soc.* 1999; **47**: 784–91.
16. Ballard CG, O'Brien J, Reichelt K, *et al.* Aromatherapy as a safe and effective treatment for the management of agitation in severe dementia: the results of a double blind, placebo controlled trial. *Journal of Clinical Psychiatry.* 2002; **63**: 553–8.
17. Holmes C, Ballard C. Aromatherapy in dementia. *Advances in Psychiatric Treatment.* 2004; **10**: 296–300.
18. McShane R, Keene J, Gedling K, *et al.* Do neuroleptic drugs hasten cognitive decline in dementia? Prospective study with necropsy follow up. *BMJ.* 1997; **314**: 266–70.
19. Kilic C, Curran HV, Noshirvani H, *et al.* Long-term effects of alprazolam on memory: a 3.5 year follow-up of agoraphobia/panic patients. *Psychological Medicine.* 1999; **29**: 225–31.
20. Tyrer P. Current problems with the benzodiazepines. In: Wheatly D, editor. *The Anxiolytic Jungle: Where Next?* Chichester: Wiley; 1990.

CHAPTER 5

Alcohol and drugs

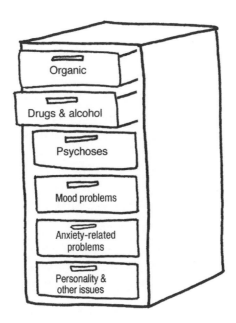

BIOLOGY OF ADDICTION

What is the biological root of our cravings? A main part of the answer lies in the brain's reward system. The pleasure centre is the general term used for the brain structures including a set of neurones found in the ventral tegmental area, which connects to the nucleus accumbens (within the limbic system) and to other areas in the prefrontal cortex. Electronic stimulation of these brain circuits have produced such bliss in rats that they have dismissed the pleasures of water, food and even the sexual advances of their fluffy acquaintances! It has been found that most abused drugs also stimulate this system.

'SOME PEOPLE TAKE DRUGS TO GET HIGH; OTHERS TAKE DRUGS TO GET BY'

These are two opposite ends of a continuum and most users of drugs and alcohol will fall somewhere between these two extremes.

Some people take drugs to get high . . .

People misuse drugs for various reasons. For those who have uncomplicated premorbid mental health who take a drug purely for pleasure, 'here and now' interventions are likely to suffice in bringing about healthy change. These interventions might involve psychological, social and possibly pharmacological support. Readiness for change issues will be addressed and 'motivational interviewing' might be employed. This is covered in Chapter 12: 'Psychological tools – promoting change in a specific area'. Conditioning is relevant here. In a situation where the drug has previously been taken one is more likely to experience craving. This 'drug compensatory conditioned response' leads to tolerance if the drug is given and withdrawal symptoms if it is not. The drug acamprosate, which reduces craving in alcohol dependence, modulates the biology of this conditioned response. It is well worth paying attention to the role of environmental 'cues' in drug use; while fighting in Vietnam many American soldiers took heroin-like drugs in order to cope with their experiences. Many became hooked but when they returned home after the war, most did not have any significant craving for the drug. They were away from the drug-taking cues (reminders/associations).[1]

In primary care we are able to employ motivational interviewing and discuss environmental cues with our patients.

In the case of problem drinking brief interventions are just as effective as long intense therapies. It has also been found that the extent of direct confrontation (as opposed to the styles employed in motivation interviewing) is predictive of continued drinking at one year.[2] Confrontational approaches can do harm.

The mnemonic **FRAMES** is used to remind us of what constitutes brief intervention.[3]

F: Feedback of risk/impairment (e.g. the fact that gamma-GT is raised suggests that alcohol is having a detrimental effect on the liver)
R: Responsibility (emphasis on their responsibility to address)
A: Advice to change (interestingly not a feature of motivational interviewing – *see* Chapter 12)
M: Menu of alternative options (the provision of literature, details of local agencies, referral options)
E: Empathy (reflective listening – *see* Chapter 11)
S: Facilitation of Self-efficacy (*see* Chapter 12 – e.g. 'confidence scale')

Others take drugs to get by . . .

Although these 'here and now' approaches are relevant to the management of all drug problems, the situation is often more complex with there being marked comorbidity in terms of formal psychiatric illness or deeply ingrained personality problems that reflect attachment issues. You will recall from Chapter 1 how these abnormal attachment patterns and behaviours are understood in terms of the characteristics of the care given in childhood. The problematic patterns of relationships which they have learnt as children are still displayed in their relationships with their current carers (usually health staff). The primary care practitioner may be the only 'permanent fixture' in the patient's life and to be effective in our management of these problems we need to have an understanding of these issues. Patients may have underlying emotionally unstable personality traits, such as:

➤ chronic feelings of emptiness
➤ intolerance of being alone – frantic efforts to avoid real or imagined abandonment
➤ a pattern of intense and unstable personal relationships characterised by alternating between extremes of idealisation and devaluation ('you are a great doctor . . . you are a sh..t doctor!')
➤ identity disturbance: persistently unstable self-image
➤ impulsivity in areas that are self-damaging
➤ sudden overwhelming outbursts of anger and destructiveness
➤ failure of **self-soothing** when faced with difficult circumstances/emotions (as they have not been able to take on and internalise good nurturing from the mother or primary care giver)
➤ recurrent suicidal behaviour or acts of self-harm
➤ affective instability (marked reactivity of immediate mood)
➤ a tendency to polarise the world into black and white, good and evil
➤ treating the body as an 'other', which can be used for gratification or attack
➤ 'perversity' – the tendency to persist in apparently self-defeating strategies when thwarted.[4]

These traits are considered further in Chapter 9. Management of these attachment issues is covered more thoroughly in Chapter 11.

Many patients will have very chaotic habits and lifestyles which provide an effective defence against underlying psychological pain and despair relating to past abuse. Having to be preoccupied with where the next 'fix' is going to come from is a useful distraction from deeper more painful psychological issues. This is why distress is often heightened when the chaos becomes under control, leading to relapse. One of my patients told me that heroin made them feel like they were 'wrapped up in cotton wool', that they felt deeply cosy and warm. This was a significant contrast to their useful feelings of emptiness and self-hate.

Substitute drugs such as methadone or buprenorphine (subutex) can bring about some containment of the individual and provide a cushion for them to face their own painful thoughts and feelings. The drug can also be considered to be a transitional object (*see* Chapter 1 – attachment theory) and provides self-soothing. It can also be viewed as a less pathological transitional object than the street drug with all its associated chaos. It can be titrated against the degree of trauma and chaos. The situation is rather like a psychological ulcer with the street drug being used as a dirty dressing or bandage. This can be changed to a prescribed clean bandage and then the wound can be gradually cleaned and debrided to allow for healthy healing.[5]

Spending on drug treatment has been shown to save money mainly through reduced criminality. The national treatment outcome research study found that for every pound the UK government spent on drug treatment, three pounds were saved![6]

There should be local arrangements for the management of alcohol and drug dependency. Remember that in alcohol dependency, sudden withdrawal without benzodiazepine cover can be life threatening. Withdrawal from opiates such as heroin is very uncomfortable but is not life threatening. We can always offer medications to reduce discomfort such as diclofenac for cramps, loperamide for diarrhoea, and prochlorperazine buccal for vomiting.

The writing of the rest of this chapter has been helped greatly by the availability of material provided by The Royal College of General Practitioners of England[7] and also by the 2003 SIGN guideline: *The Management of Harmful Drinking and Alcohol Dependence in Primary Care*.[8]

ASSESSMENT OF SUBSTANCE MISUSE

In primary care we should at the very least be able to offer the basics of assessment and advice concerning harm reduction. This may need to take place over a number of appointment slots. We'll now take a look at what this involves.

History

Drug behaviour

➤ What? (alcohol, cannabis, amphetamine, heroin, cocaine, ecstasy etc). Drug users may refer to a 'gram' of street heroin or may use 'teenths' (sixteenths) of an ounce in describing their use. 'Half a teenth' is just less than a 'gram'.
➤ When? (eye-opener first thing in the morning to prevent withdrawal symptoms)
➤ How? (mode of use – inject or smoke)
➤ Why? (self-medication for other mental health difficulties)

Drug dependence syndrome

Establish whether this is a drug dependence syndrome. This is considered to be present when three or more of the following are present:

➤ strong desire or compulsion to use the drug
➤ difficulty controlling the use of the drug
➤ withdrawal symptoms when the use of the drug is ceased (e.g. anxiety, tremors, sweating in the case of alcohol)
➤ tolerance (having to use more of the drug to obtain the same effect)
➤ continued use of the drug despite harmful consequences.

Remember the diagnostic hierarchy (see Chapter 3)

Perform a systems review for physical health and also establish whether there are any psychotic features, mood disturbance, anxiety issues and eating disorder related problems. It might be helpful to incorporate some of the screening questions from the subsequent chapters.

Social history

Include details of dependent children as drug misuse may impact on the quality of parenting due to reduced availability both from a supervisory and emotional point of view. Hence a potential risk of accidents, neglect, emotional deprivation, ingestion of parent's drugs and poverty.

ICE

Address the Ideas, Concerns and Expectations of the patient.

Physical examination, screening for drug use and investigations

Include examination of injecting sites, blood pressure and peak flow if the drug is being smoked.

Urine (or mouth swab) should always be sent to the laboratory to confirm drug use before initiating treatment. Screening should be continued during the course of treatment in order to monitor treatment. Treatment should not be withdrawn because of subsequent test results indicating continued illicit drug use; rather these results should be used as an adjunct to treatment and not used punitively.

Perform relevant investigations as indicated by the history and examination.

Harm reduction advice

Provide advice about local needle exchanges and safer injecting such as that in Part Four, Patient resources.

Discuss sexual health, including the following.
➤ Menstrual periods may be absent or irregular but pregnancy is still possible.
➤ Limit number of sexual partners.
➤ Ideally be monogamous with current partner.
➤ To help prevent pregnancy use effective contraception as well as condoms.
➤ Use condoms for sexually transmitted infection (STI) prevention.

MANAGEMENT
Blood-borne viruses
Encourage the patient to have blood taken for hepatitis and HIV serology and to have vaccination against hepatitis B.

Hepatitis B
This is transmitted as a result of blood-to-blood contact including the sharing of blood contaminated needles and other injecting equipment.

Incubation period is six weeks to six months with an average of three months.

In adults about 30% of acute infections result in jaundice and many cases are not diagnosed.

It is unwise to delay administration of the first dose of vaccine while awaiting serology test results as co-infection with hepatitis A or B significantly worsens the morbidity and mortality associated with hepatitis C. If a positive result for A or B is then obtained, it can be discussed with the patient and immunisation discontinued. It is always best practice to confirm with serology, but there is no need to wait.

Hepatitis B vaccine
Accelerated regimens are now recommended for drug users, i.e. doses are given at Days 0, 7 and 21 with a booster at 12 months. This may improve completion rates over slower vaccination regimes, especially if the patient may leave before completing.

Vaccination is recommended for intravenous drug users not already infected or immune, and for close household contacts, particularly sexual partners and children.

Hepatitis A vaccination is also recommended for injecting drug users but separate vaccinations appear superior to the combined vaccine.

Hepatitis C

The virus may be contracted by sharing needles and syringes. It is mainly transmitted by direct blood-borne contact. Transmission by the sexual route is rare but may be increasing.

An initial antibody test will indicate whether or not he or she has been infected.

Twenty to fifty per cent of people will clear the virus at the acute stage. Of the other remaining people, three-quarters will go on to have a chronic syndrome with tiredness and lethargy, a proportion will go on to develop liver disease and cirrhosis and a minority will have potentially fatal hepatic complications, such as liver cancer. Prognosis is worse in older patients, males, and co-infection with other types of hepatitis or HIV. Some patients, however, are asymptomatic, with normal liver function blood test results, but this does not mean that their liver is not damaged and continuing to be damaged.

In order to establish if the virus is still present and to diagnose the extent of the disease further specialist tests are required. A polymerase chain reaction (PCR) test for hepatitis C will identify if there is a circulating virus. The amount of virus (viral load) and the genotype of the virus can also be tested. Treatment for hepatitis C has improved and referral to a liver specialist or infectious diseases unit for assessment is recommended.

Hepatitis C positive patients should be advised to eat a healthy diet and strongly advised to refrain from all alcohol. They should take particular caution to avoid others coming into contact with their blood, never share injecting equipment and never share used toothbrushes or razors. There is a very small risk of transmission due to sexual intercourse, so condoms should be used.

Opiate withdrawal symptoms

It is common for patients awaiting treatment to request medication such as weak opioids (e.g. dihydrocodeine) but these should be declined because:
➤ these tablets need to be taken frequently and can therefore reinforce drug taking behaviour
➤ dihydrocodeine is more of a euphoriant than methadone or buprenorphine.

Symptoms and signs of opiate withdrawal include:
➤ **symptoms**: anorexia, nausea, abdominal pain, hot and cold flushes, joint pains, insomnia, cramps, craving
➤ **signs**: restlessness, yawning, sweating, runny nose and eyes, dilated pupils, muscle twitching, vomiting, and diarrhoea.

Some patients may be able to go 24 hours between using, while for others, there may be a need to use four- to six-hourly to prevent withdrawals. Typically the time of last dose to onset of withdrawals decreases with a longer history of drug use.

Occasionally, prescribing symptomatic treatment may be appropriate as outlined in Table 5.1.

TABLE 5.1 Symptomatic treatment for opiate withdrawal

Symptom	Drug	Dose
Stomach cramps	Buscopan	10–20 mg eight-hourly
Diarrhoea	Loperamide	2 mg, max eight-daily
Musculoskeletal pain	Ibuprofen	200–400 mg six- to eight-hourly

Treatment planning

There is good evidence that maintenance treatment with a replacement opioid such as methadone or buprenorphine reduces the risk of death, reduces injecting, illicit drug use, blood-borne-virus risk behaviour, crime, and improves physical and mental health.

Though it is impossible to be completely prescriptive about who is and who is not suitable for primary care treatment, a wide range of patients can be successfully managed in primary care, though patients with serious psychological or psychiatric, social or medical problems may be better served by specialist services.

Maintenance prescribing, often within a shared care framework and in accordance with national and local guidelines, is a highly effective treatment.

ALCOHOL PROBLEMS

Alcohol use disorders identification test C (AUDIT C)

In primary care it is important to identify those people who could be physically or emotionally at risk from their drinking habits, not just those who are dependent. The AUDIT C (*see* Appendix 1: Alcohol questionnaires) is an effective brief screening test for problem drinking and dependency. It will detect 75% of problem drinkers.[9] Specificity is low, however, and there is no substitute for a decent clinical chat to separate the wheat from the chaff or perhaps I should say the mice from the fluff – remember a sensitive screening tool such as the AUDIT C is rather like a sensitive mouse trap: it is very effective at trapping most of the mice but unfortunately it will trap lots of fluff, dust and spiders as well!

If the score is eight or more indicating possible hazardous use, we can then use the CAGE questionnaire (*see* Appendix 1) which, when used alone, is a validated screening test for alcohol abuse and dependence.[10]

The combination of CAGE questionnaire, mean corpuscular volume (MCV) – can be raised with high alcohol consumption – and gamma-glutamyl transferase (GGT), a liver enzyme that can be raised with high alcohol consumption, will detect about 75% of people with an alcohol problem.

A unit of alcohol is approximately a single short, glass of wine or half a pint of beer.

Use of over 21 units per week for men and over 14 units per week for women can be harmful with risk of physical harm (e.g. liver disease, gastrointestinal haemorrhage), psychological harm (e.g. depressed mood and anxiety due to alcohol) or social harm (e.g. loss of job, relationship difficulties).

Problem drinking (not dependent)

There is good evidence to support brief nonspecialist intervention in managing problem drinking. Assessing intake, giving advice on reducing consumption and 'motivational interviewing' have been found to be effective in bringing about significant reductions in alcohol consumption. Stages of change and motivational interviewing will be discussed in Chapter 12. Motivational interviewing techniques are a refreshing and effective way of leading the individual to specify all the reasons they wish to change and why change is important to them.

We can then discuss goals with our patients after informing them of acceptable levels of drinking. In Part Four there is an advice sheet – 'advice for problem drinkers'. This contains suitable targets for males and females and advice on how to reach target. These tips could form the basis of initial goal setting.

Alcohol dependency

Sudden cessation of alcohol in the dependent can be life threatening. Delirium tremens ('the DTs') occurs 48–72 hours or more after the last drink. Delirium (acute confusion) with agitation, visual and auditory hallucinations, and paranoia can occur. There are associated complications of convulsions, hyperthermia, dehydration, and blood biochemical imbalance which can be life threatening. This is a medical emergency and medical hospital admission is required. It is easy to forget that alcohol withdrawal could be the cause of acute confusion. The person might not even smell of alcohol as there can be a delay of a few days before the symptoms show themselves.

Detoxification in hospital

Withdrawal should take place in hospital in the following circumstances:
- history of withdrawal seizures
- signs of delirium
- severe vomiting
- risk of suicide
- lack of social support
- severe dependence coupled with unwillingness to be seen daily
- failure of home assisted withdrawal
- uncontrollable withdrawal symptoms
- acute physical illness
- multiple drug misuse
- home environment unsupportive of abstinence.[8]

Detoxification in the community

For those with alcohol dependence syndrome, detoxification at home can be considered when the individual is motivated to stop drinking and when there is adequate social support. The patient should be seen daily and therefore a team approach is likely to be necessary. Before embarking on a home detoxification consider the following risks:
- accident from over-sedation
- deliberate overdose of prescribed drugs
- dependence on prescribed drugs
- physical complications of withdrawal (e.g. convulsions).

TABLE 5.2 Chlordiazepoxide 10 mg reducing regime[7]

	First thing Number of tablets	12 noon Number of tablets	6 pm Number of tablets	Bedtime Number of tablets
Day 1	None	3	3	3
Day 2	2	2	2	3
Day 3	2	1	1	2
Day 4	1	1	None	2
Day 5	None	1	None	1

Table 5.2 provides a reducing medication regime using chlordiazepoxide (Librium) 10 mg tablets. The drug stimulates the same brain receptor as alcohol (the GABA receptor) and with a reducing dose helps to reduce the

withdrawal symptoms of headache, nausea, vomiting, sweating and tremor, and helps to prevent convulsions.

Also prescribe the oral vitamin B preparation of thiamine 50 mg twice daily for three weeks to prevent Wernicke's encephalopathy.

Patients 'at risk' of developing Wernicke's encephalopathy (those who are malnourished or with diarrhoea, vomiting, physical illness, weight loss) should receive parenteral vitamin supplementation during detoxification. There is a very small risk of anaphylaxis with parenteral vitamin supplementation. Intramuscular Pabrinex should be given where there are facilities for treating anaphylactic reactions such as in the GP surgery, emergency department, outpatient clinic or day hospital. One pair of ampoules should be administered daily for three days.[7]

Signs of possible Wernicke-Korsakov syndrome include confusion, ataxia, ophthalmoplegia, nystagmus, memory disturbance, hypothermia, hypotension and coma. Any patient who presents with unexplained neurological symptoms or signs during detoxification should be referred for specialist assessment for urgent treatment.

Abstinence should be the short-term goal, while not ruling out subsequent controlled drinking.

Assisting with abstinence from alcohol

The following may help with abstinence.
➤ Enlist the support of family and friends. Encourage the patient to be open with the 'significant others' in his or her life about vulnerability to relapse and the need for assistance in dealing with particular environmental cues that are likely to enhance cravings. The patient may wish to bring a family member or friend along to consultations to help with planning strategies.
➤ Refer to local alcohol services, e.g. Alcoholics Anonymous (AA).
➤ Consider specific pharmacotherapy.

There is much evidence in support of the efficacy and cost effectiveness of medications for relapse prevention.[11]

Acamprosate is believed to act by modulating disturbance in the gamma-aminobutyric acid/glutamate system associated with alcohol dependence and the drug compensatory conditioned response. It is a safe drug with few unwanted side-effects, and is not liable to misuse. Its value is in the first months after detoxification. Acamprosate is not effective in all patients so its efficacy should be assessed at regular appointments, and the drug withdrawn if there has not been a major reduction in drinking. Where it appears to be effective, good practice suggests prescribing for 6–12 months.

Disulfiram acts as a deterrent. If taken regularly there is an unpleasant reaction when alcohol is consumed. It has unwanted effects in some patients, and carries special warnings. If used, it should be offered for six months in the first instance, with regular review. Supervision is agreed by the patient to increase the likelihood that the medication is taken even at times of ambivalence. Disulfiram supervision may be undertaken by the spouse, healthcare or support worker, or the workplace representative if appropriate.

➤ Always accompany pharmacotherapy with alcohol-focused counselling.
➤ Initiate active intervention if other psychiatric problems persist.
➤ Give ongoing support.[7]

Relapse

The process of recovery is likely to involve several relapses. Carry on with a non-confrontational approach.

REFERENCES

1. Robins LN, Helzer JE, Davis DH. Narcotic use in Southeast Asia and afterward. An interview study of 898 Vietnam returnees. *Arch Gen Psychiatry.* 1975; **32**: 955–61.
2. Miller W, *et al.* Enhancing motivation to change in problem drinking: a controlled comparison of two therapist styles. *J Consult Clin Psychol.* 1993; **61**: 455–61.
3. Bien TH, Miller WR, Tonigan JS. Brief interventions for alcohol problems: a review. *Addiction.* 1993; **88**(3): 315–35.
4. Holmes J. Psychotherapeutic approaches to the management of severe personality disorder in general psychiatric settings. *CPD Bulletin Psychiatry.* 1999; **1**(2): 35–41.
5. Lecture; Psychotherapy of the Addiction. Vanessa J Griffiths, Consultant Clinical Psychologist, Cornwall Drug and Alcohol Team.
6. Gossop M, Marsden J, Stewart D, *et al.* The National Treatment Outcome Research Study (NTORS): 4–5 year follow-up results. *Addiction.* 2003; **98**: 291–303.
7. www.rcgp.org.uk
8. Scottish Intercollegiate Guidelines Network. *The Management of Harmful Drinking and Alcohol Dependence in Primary Care: A National Clinical Guideline.* Edinburgh; SIGN: 2003 (SIGN Guideline 74). [cited 1 February 2008]. Available at: www.sign.ac.uk/guidelines/fulltext/74/index.html
9. Bush K, Kivlahan DR, McDonell MB, *et al.* The AUDIT alcohol consumption questions (AUDIT-C): an effective brief screening test for problem drinking. *Arch Intern Med.* 1998; **158**: 1789–95.
10. Ewing JA. Detecting alcoholism. The CAGE questionnaire. *JAMA.* 1984; **252**(14): 1905–7.
11. Garbutt JC, West SL, Carey TS, *et al.* Pharmacological treatment of alcohol dependence: a review of the evidence. *JAMA.* 1999; **281**(14): 1318–25.

CHAPTER 6

Psychosis

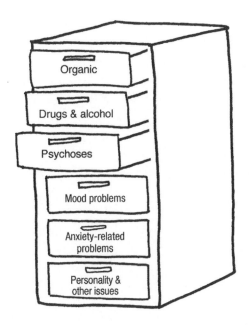

A person is psychotic if they have lost touch with reality. These conditions are characterised by delusions and hallucinations. A delusion is a firmly held false belief out of keeping with the individual's culture. A hallucination is a perception without a stimulus – the individual may hear, see, smell, taste or touch something that is not actually present.

In this chapter I hope to introduce some interesting concepts about the psychoses and useful consultation questions. When considering diagnosis we need to remember that someone with psychotic symptoms may have an organic or drug-related problem and might therefore be more appropriately positioned in a more elevated hierarchical position. Although psychosis in mania and depression is dealt with in the next chapter the assessment questions highlighted below can usefully be applied to any psychotic presentation.

A SPECTRUM OF RELATED CONDITIONS?

'Psychosis' refers to a real 'mixed bag' of problems. We can keep it simple by remembering the 'stress-vulnerability' framework discussed in Chapters 1 and 2. Assessment questions really help us to uncover the symptomatology that frequently exists with psychotic illness but the symptoms uncovered give us no clues as to the cause of the problems and the likely outcome for the individual we are working with. There may be a predisposition relating to genetics or obstetric complications. There seems to be growing acceptance of the idea that a number of states are genetically related and fall somewhere on a 'schizophrenia spectrum'. For some, the presence or absence of physical (e.g. illicit drugs) or emotional stressors will determine whether frank psychotic symptoms of delusions and hallucinations will emerge. It is possible that some individuals do not become psychotic but remain eccentric with odd thinking, behaviour and affect. The movement of 'Schizotypal Personality Disorder' from the personality disorder section of the ICD-10 to the 'Schizophrenia, schizotypal and delusional disorders' section reflects the acceptance of a 'spectrum' of genetically related conditions.

'Positive' symptoms

'Positive' symptoms are hallucinations and delusions. When the onset is abrupt, they tend to respond well to medication treatments so maybe there is something positive about them after all. I remember a patient whose illness had led her to become extremely isolated socially. The only positive thing she could identify in her life was her 'friendly voice'. It seemed to provide her with company and reassurance and was truly a 'positive' psychotic symptom. The problem was that by eradicating the nasty voices, treatment left her grieving for the nice one which also left her. On balance, her life did improve in the long run.

Many of us will remember the phrase 'first rank symptoms' of schizophrenia. Some of the assessment questions outlined below try to uncover these 'positive' symptoms. These were given importance by Kurt Schneider in 1959. The reason we readily accepted his ideas was probably because he was a German without Nazi sympathies. He introduced the concept of 'loss of ego boundaries'. He felt that his first rank symptoms (passivity, thought interference, delusions of control, thought broadcast, third person auditory hallucinations, commentary hallucinations, delusional perception*) were evidence of loss of ego boundaries, i.e. not knowing when 'I' ends and 'not I' begins. I find this interesting as I have an interest in meditation. Many people

---

* Delusional perception – a delusional interpretation of a perception, e.g. the fact that the cup is on the table means that I am a sheep!

report that the pleasant feelings of meditation are associated with an expansive experience where one feels at one with the surroundings. Schneider may well have considered me to have been severely ill because of my experiences. In any case, I do think it is useful to have had these common symptoms described to us. It is a shame that they have no predictive value in determining outcome or the course of someone's illness. Twin studies have shown that Schneider's first rank symptoms define a form of schizophrenia with the least evidence of inheritance. These first rank symptoms are still regarded as being important in making a diagnosis of schizophrenia – *see* the ICD-10 criteria below.

'Negative' symptoms

Timothy Crow (1980) described type I and type II schizophrenia. Type I is characterised by acute onset, positive symptoms, normal brain ventricles and good response to medication and was thought to be due to an increase in the activity of the neurotransmitter dopamine. Type II had a more insidious onset with enlarged ventricles and a poor response to medication and a deteriorating course. 'Negative' symptoms are listed in ICD-10 criteria below. The truth is that we can have both positive and negative symptoms. The newer 'atypical' antipsychotic medications target the negative symptoms better by acting on a number of receptors, bringing about change in a number of neurotransmitter systems. Patients can develop secondary negative symptoms – a side-effect of antipsychotic medication and most likely in first generation antipsychotics.

ICD-10 criteria for the diagnosis of schizophrenia

Symptoms must be present for most of the time during an episode of psychotic illness lasting for at least one month (or at some time during most of the days).

At least one of the following must be present:

1   thought echo, thought insertion or withdrawal, or thought broadcasting
2   delusions of control, influence or passivity, clearly referred to body or limb movements or specific thoughts, actions or sensations, delusional perception
3   hallucinatory voices giving a running commentary on the patient's behaviour, or discussing the patient among themselves, or other types of hallucinatory voices coming from some part of the body
4   persistent delusions of other kinds that are culturally inappropriate and completely impossible.

Or at least two of the following:

1 persistent hallucinations in any modality, when occurring every day for at least one month, when accompanied by delusions (which may be fleeting or half formed) without clear affective content or when accompanied by persistent overvalued ideas
2 neologising, breaks or interpolations in the train of thought, resulting in incoherence or irrelevant speech
3 catatonic behaviour, such as excitement, posturing or waxy flexibility, mutism and stupor
4 'negative' symptoms such as marked apathy, paucity of speech and blunting or incongruity of emotional responses (it must be clear that these are not due to depression or to neuroleptic medication).

Neuro-developmental model

As far back as 1896 some sort of developmental problem was being considered. At that time Emil Kraeplin described 'Dementia Praecox', a state of steady decline in mental functioning and where for some cases it was significant that from childhood 'a degree of psychic weakness existed'. Bleuler invented the label 'schizophrenia' in 1911 and talked about early character anomalies 'which can be demonstrated by careful case histories in more than half the individuals who become schizophrenic'. He described a tendency to seclusion, withdrawal, irritability and inability to play with other children. This developmental way of thinking was waylaid in England by an anti-establishment movement and a wish not to be associated in any way with the Nazis, hence the adoption of Schneider's ideas. However, now there is growing support for a neuro-developmental model with behavioural, cognitive and motor differences being found in children who develop psychoses. Functional brain imaging used to determine brain activity in hallucinators by looking at cerebral blood flow has shown evidence of brain 'wiring' problems and inner speech being misattributed to an external source. There has also been the research associating obstetric complications, enlarged ventricles, negative symptoms and worse outcome. More recently there has been interest in the role of glial cells in psychosis. Glial cells in the brain provide a scaffolding around which cortical cells migrate. These cortical nerve cells (neurons) undergo a maturation process in adolescence and there is a 'pruning' activity at this time. Perhaps there is a genetic defect in controlling this activity for some people who develop psychosis. Many people do not realise that the brain is not 'matured' until the early 20s. Imagine what effects the taking of illicit drugs might have on this developing system. There must surely be a risk to the developing personality as well as the possibility of illness being precipitated.

ASSESSMENT

Individuals with psychosis may have very little insight into their problem. This means that there may be a failure to appreciate that symptoms are not real or caused by illness. They may resent the fuss that is being made and may believe there is a conspiracy against them. They can be angry or fearful. Questioning needs to be handled sensitively in order to avoid confrontation. Non-specialists may have little experience in talking to psychotic people. We may find ourselves assessing someone suffering their first psychotic episode or taking part in an assessment which may lead to compulsory hospital admission. Observing and listening may give you all the information you need. There are many assessment questions and I am sure it is not necessary to remember them all. Committing some of them to memory or to a crib sheet may help if there is silence or if you feel the need to assess more deeply.

Breaking the ice

➤ 'I gather your (mum) is worried about you. I wonder why that is? [*pause*]' *or* 'Do you know why this is?'

This question is a useful way of getting started. It can helpfully take the heat out of a situation. It then allows us to use our open questions to explore what the patient has been experiencing or what significant others may have noticed about them.

We may then need to close down our questioning style.

Some useful screening questions

➤ 'Do you hear voices when no one is around? What do they say?'
➤ 'Do you ever think that people are talking or gossiping about you, maybe even thinking about trying to get you?'
➤ 'Do you ever think that somehow people can pick up on what you are thinking or can manipulate what you are thinking?'[1]

Assessing perception – hallucination: a perception without stimulus

Visual, olfactory (smell) or gustatory (taste) hallucinations should make you consider an organic cause.

➤ 'Does your imagination ever play tricks on you?'
➤ 'Do you ever get the feeling that there is something odd going on that you cannot explain?'
➤ 'Is there anything unusual about the way things look or sound, or smell, or taste?'

Auditory hallucinations
➤ 'Do you ever hear something that you find difficult to account for?' . . .
'Can you give me an example?' *If the patient does not seem to understand the question*: 'Sometimes people hear things when there is nothing actually there to explain it, like a voice calling their name.'
➤ 'Do the voices come from inside or outside your head?'
➤ 'How many voices do you hear?'
➤ 'Do they ever comment on your actions?'
➤ 'Do they talk about you?' (*third person hallucinations*)
➤ 'Do they talk to you?' (*second person hallucinations*)
➤ 'Do they ever tell you what to do?' (*command hallucinations*)
➤ 'Do you have to obey them?' (*assessing risk to self or others*)

Assessing thought – delusion: firmly held false beliefs out of keeping with the individual's culture
➤ 'Is there any subject you often get into arguments with others about?'
➤ 'Is there any force or power other than yourself trying to take control of you?' (*somatic passivity*)
➤ 'Is any person or group of people trying to harm you?'
➤ 'Does the TV or radio talk about you?' (*delusions of reference*)
➤ 'Do you see any special meaning for yourself in everyday objects?' (*delusions of reference*)
➤ 'Does the world around you seem to have changed in a way that is difficult to explain?' (*delusional mood*)

Assessing thought – thought block
➤ 'Do you ever experience your thoughts stopping quite unexpectedly so that there are none left in your mind, even when your thoughts were flowing freely before?'

Assessing thought – thought interference
➤ 'Does anything interfere with your thoughts in any way?'
➤ 'Are you in full control of your thoughts?'
➤ 'Are thoughts put into your head which you know are not your own?' (*thought insertion*) . . . 'How do you know they are not your own?' . . . 'Where do they come from?'
➤ 'Do you ever hear your thoughts spoken aloud?' (*thought broadcast*)
➤ 'Do you ever hear your thoughts repeated in your head?' (*thought echo*)
➤ 'Do you ever experience thoughts being taken out of your head, as if some external person or force is removing them?' (*thought withdrawal*)

BIOLOGICAL TREATMENTS

It has been known for many years that excessive dopamine transmission in the brain's mesolimbic system plays a key role in psychosis. The clinical efficacy of first generation antipsychotics (often called 'typical' antipsychotics) is closely correlated to their ability to block dopamine. The second generation drugs ('atypical' antipsychotics) have a broader action, acting on additional brain receptors. With the exception of clozapine which seems superior in treatment resistant cases, there is no convincing evidence that the newer drugs are more effective at treating psychosis. Though they are less liable to bring about extrapyramidal (parkinsonian) side-effects of stiffness and tremor, they can have significant side-effects of their own as set out below.

Common side-effects of first generation antipsychotics

➤ Extrapyramidal effects:
  – dystonia
  – pseudoparkinsonism
  – akathisia (an unpleasant subjective sensation of 'inner' restlessness that manifests itself with an inability to sit still or remain motionless)
  – tardive dyskinesia (characterised by repetitive, involuntary, purposeless movements. Features of the disorder may include grimacing, tongue protrusion, lip smacking, puckering and pursing, and rapid eye blinking. Rapid movements of the arms, legs and trunk may also occur. Involuntary movements of the fingers may appear as though the patient is playing an invisible guitar or piano).
➤ Sedation.
➤ Hyperprolactinaemia.
➤ Reduced seizure threshold.
➤ Postural hypotension.
➤ Anticholinergic effects:
  – Blurred vision
  – Dry mouth
  – Urinary retention.
➤ Neuroleptic malignant syndrome.
  (Neuroleptic malignant syndrome is a life-threatening, neurological disorder most often caused by an adverse reaction to neuroleptic or antipsychotic drugs. Symptoms include high fever, sweating, unstable blood pressure, stupor, muscular rigidity, and autonomic dysfunction.)
➤ Weight gain.
➤ Sexual dysfunction.
➤ Cardiotoxicity.

Common side effects of second generation antipsychotics

➤ Olanzapine: weight gain; sedation; glucose intolerance and diabetes mellitus; hypotension.
➤ Risperidone: hyperprolactinaemia; hypotension; extrapyramidal side-effects at higher doses; sexual dysfunction.
➤ Amisulpiride: hyperprolactinaemia; insomnia; extrapyramidal effects.
➤ Quetiapine: hypotension; dyspepsia; drowsiness.
➤ Clozapine: sedation; hypersalivation; constipation; reduced seizure threshold; hypotension and hypertension; tachycardia; pyrexia; weight gain; glucose intolerance and diabetes mellitus; nocturnal enuresis. Also rare but serious haematological side-effects requiring blood monitoring.

PSYCHOSOCIAL TREATMENTS

We should also be aware of the family/home dynamics; the levels of criticism, hostility and over-involvement. We discussed this issue of 'expressed emotion' in Chapter 1. It must be a very difficult balance to get right when a loved one develops psychosis. It would be natural to be emotionally charged. Modifying emotional responses might require the assistance of a professional trained in family interventions that have been proven to reduce relapse rates. Cognitive behaviour therapy (CBT) approaches can be used to reduce the intensity and frequency of psychotic experiences.

These approaches can make a substantial difference to residual symptoms. Both distraction and focusing approaches have been studied. Distraction might involve using a personal stereo or reading out loud to make the hallucinatory voices less distressing. Focusing involves graded exposure of the individual to the voices, anxiety management, exploration of beliefs and meanings associated with the voices and modifying the beliefs to reduce the negative impact they have. Focusing approaches have had a better effect on self-esteem. CBT has also been utilised for delusions. The concept that a belief is either shakeable or unshakeable (i.e. a delusion) is somewhat 'black and white'. In truth, there will be varying degrees of certainty with which a belief is held by an individual and the process of CBT will allow the person to look at evidence for and against the thoughts they have with a view to getting a more balanced view of circumstances.

GENERAL HEALTHCARE NEEDS

People with mental health problems are less likely to access the physical care they need. Having a register of patients with significant mental health problems and carrying out regular health reviews will help to prevent future ill health. Some of the medications used will predispose the person to weight gain and diabetes. Some medications can cause cardiac arrhythmias. Male patients may be distressed by medication induced impotence or the growing of breast tissue (gynaecomastia). The patient may find it easier to discuss these issues with the non-specialist who may have known them for a long time. Once a problem has been identified, medications can be changed to better suit the individual.

OUTCOME

More than 80% of patients with their first episode of psychosis will recover, although less than 20% will never have another episode.[2] Rather like a gut ulcer there is a good chance of recovery but for many there will be an ongoing vulnerability to future inflammation; a large number of people will have just a few relapses with good functional recovery. Poor premorbid adjustment, a slow insidious onset, and a long duration of untreated psychosis – together with prominent negative symptoms – tend to be associated with a worse prognosis.[3] An acute onset, an obvious psychosocial precipitant, and good premorbid adjustment all improve the prognosis.

IMPROVING SOMEONE'S CHANCES

Early diagnosis and treatment leads to significantly improved recovery and outcome in psychosis – don't delay!

When an adolescent or young adult presents with persistent changes in functioning, behaviour or personality consider psychotic illness or psychotic prodrome in your differential diagnosis.

The prodromal (early) symptoms of first episode schizophrenia and the childhood characteristics of individuals who later develop these 'schizophrenia spectrum disorders' can have considerable overlap and include:

➤ **passivity** (waiting passively for instructions; rarely taking initiative; spontaneous activity rare; reduced drive, energy and motivation)
➤ **being withdrawn**
➤ **nervousness, social anxiety, hypersensitivity to criticism**
➤ **disciplinary problems, antisocial behaviour**
➤ **peculiarity, odd behaviour**
➤ **flat affect** (seldom laughing or smiling; no reaction when praised or encouraged).[4]

The early identification of symptoms in severe mental illness is important. Early intervention may improve outcome and lessen the period of distressing uncertainty experienced by families and sufferers.

Although these characteristics form part of normal adolescence for some children, teachers are in a unique position to identify those who are behaviourally distinct from their peers. These combined behaviours, when identified by teachers, have been shown to be sensitive and specific predictors of future illness. It would therefore seem sensible to obtain information from teachers when concern is raised over a child's well-being. It is possible that targeting such individuals with work on coping strategies/resilience building may help reduce the risk of future frank psychosis.

REFERENCES

1. Picchioni MM, Murray RM. Schizophrenia. *BMJ.* 2007; **335**: 91–5.
2. Robinson D, Woerner MG, Alvir JMJ, *et al.* Predictors of relapse following response from a first episode of schizophrenia or schizoaffective disorder. *Arch Gen Psychiatry.* 1999; **56**: 241–7.
3. Perkins DO, Hongbin G, Boteva K, *et al.* Relationship between duration of untreated psychosis and outcome in first-episode schizophrenia: a critical review and meta-analysis. *Am J Psychiatry.* 2005; **162**: 1785–804.
4. Morris M, MacPherson R. Childhood 'risk characteristics' and the schizophrenia spectrum prodrome. *Ir J Psych Med.* 2001; **18**(2): 72–4.

CHAPTER 7

Mood problems

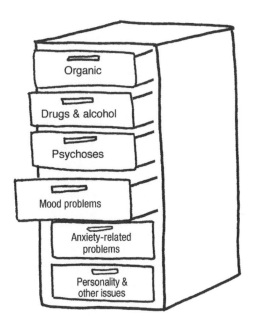

LOW MOOD

Background considerations

➤ At any given time 4–5% of the population are suffering from severe depression and 95% of these will be treated in primary care.

➤ Half the patients consulting with depression in general practice do not have their depression recognised.

➤ Consequences can be great with disorder predisposing to the development of physical ill health such as coronary artery disease and reduced bone density as well as having great psychosocial impact.

➤ In addition to effective medication treatments for major depression and dysthymia (persistent low mood not meeting the criteria for major depression), there are a number of brief psychological approaches that can be effectively applied in the general practice setting, irrespective of the severity of depressed mood.

➤ 60% of clinically depressed people respond to the first antidepressant tried (vs. 30% placebo).
➤ The average length of an untreated episode of clinical depression is eight months.

Just as psychotic problems are becoming the 'bread and butter' of the specialist services, low mood problems are becoming the 'bread and butter' of primary care. But isn't bread getting complicated these days? There seems to be numerous diagnostic labels applied to low mood-depression problems. In this chapter I am aiming to remove the confusion brought about by the differing terminology used by the classificatory systems.

We will see that it is very useful to simply focus our attention on whether the depressed mood is 'syndromal' (stuck down over time) or not. If it is, we can consider offering medication treatment. And we can use psychosocial management options for both syndromal and non-syndromal presentations.

Case study
To help us explore the recognition, assessment and management of low mood we will consider the case of a 47-year-old woman. Her mother died six months ago and she is divorcing her husband.

Getting depression on the consultation agenda
Our consultation style will have bearing on this. Giving eye contact, interrupting less, and appearing unhurried (i.e. good acting!) will increase recognition of depression by health professionals.

Where low mood is suspected for at-risk patients, such as those with chronic diseases, we can use a two-question screening instrument.
➤ 'During the past month, have you been bothered by:
  – feeling down, depressed or hopeless?
  – feeling little interest or pleasure in doing things?'

This has a sensitivity of 96% and a specificity of 57% for diagnosing major depression (clinical depression).[1,2] A 'yes' answer to either of these questions (both taken from the DSM-IV criteria for 'major depression'[3] (clinical depression) will need to prompt further assessment as there will be a lot of false positives; this sensitive test like the mouse trap is described in Chapter 7.

Is this low mood 'syndromal'?
For practical purposes I classify low mood problems into those that are likely to be antidepressant responsive and those that are not. To be responsive to

medication the low mood needs to be 'syndromal', i.e. it needs to be stuck down over time – persistently and pervasively low.

If she has answered yes to either or both of the above questions ask her:

> 'Over the last two weeks, how much of the time have you been feeling like this . . .
> . . . have you been feeling like it for less than half the days or more than half the days?'

If she has been feeling like this for more than half the days then her low mood can be considered to be syndromal. She will journey through her own grieving process in her own time. However, a persistent and pervasive low mood can interfere with normal adjustment and prevent normal grieving. Under normal circumstances, when a person is adjusting to change, social stress or to a loss, there is a recognisable lift in mood when the mind is distracted from difficulties. If her mood remains at a lower ebb without her getting her usual level of enjoyment from her activities, her mood can be considered to be pervasively low.

Start preparing a foundation for treatment by exploring what she usually enjoys. Encourage her to elaborate by enquiring about what she does, where she does it and what other people are involved.

Find out about functional impairment:

> 'With the way you have been feeling how difficult has it been for you to do your work, take care of things at home, or get along with other people?'

Antidepressants are likely to be helpful if she is functionally impaired and has at least five depressive features,[4,5] with at least one from the two questions above and the others from the list below (taken from the DSM-IV criteria). If this is the case she has 'major depression'.

If she is persistently and pervasively low with functional impairment yet does not have the five features it is better to defer treatment with antidepressants. Monitor and employ psychological interventions. Given that patients with more chronic 'low grade' forms of depression such as dysthymia may benefit from antidepressants, consider the use of antidepressants if there is no improvement over one to two months.[6–8]

Other features of depression
➤ Significant weight loss or gain (more than 5% change in one month) or an increase or decrease in appetite nearly every day.

➤ Insomnia or hypersomnia nearly every day.
➤ Psychomotor agitation or retardation nearly every day (observable by others).
➤ Fatigue or loss of energy nearly every day.
➤ Feelings of worthlessness or excessive or inappropriate guilt (which may be delusional) nearly every day (not merely self-reproach about being sick).
➤ Diminished ability to think or concentrate, or indecisiveness, nearly every day.
➤ Recurrent thoughts of death (not just fear of dying), recurrent suicidal ideation without a specific plan or a suicide attempt or a specific plan for committing suicide.

Psychological issues

Suicidality

Asking about suicide will not increase the risk. You may need to broach the subject gently.

> 'How do you see the future?'
> 'Has life seemed quite hopeless?'
> 'Can you see any future?'
> 'Have you given up or does there still seem some reason for trying?'
> 'Have you felt that life wasn't worth living?'
> 'Did you ever feel like ending it all?'
> 'What did you think you might do?'

Thinking style

Is there a negative pattern of thinking that may have contributed to the development of her depression or maintenance of her low mood? Is she having negative thoughts that may not be fully justified? Does she recognise/understand this? You could discuss the thinking errors in Chapter 2 to see if she finds any similarities with her own cognitive style.

Loss

Can she tell you about how she has felt since the loss of her mother and marital relationship?

Social issues

Presence or absence of support and a confidant(e)

Is she satisfied with her current social situation? This is more important than whether she is simply isolated or not.

Ongoing stressors

How is the divorce progressing? Uncertainty is stressful. Are there any other factors? Has she got a strategy or plan to deal with the problems or does she feel hopeless and unable to cope?

Remember the hierarchy

Thyroid disorder; early menopause; prescribed medicines; alcohol and illicit drugs. Screen for psychosis – *see* Chapter 6.

Screen for mania:

> 'Has there ever been a period of at least four days when you were so happy or excited that you got into trouble, or your family or friends worried about it?'

Screen for anxiety. It is common for anxiety to coexist with depression. Ask about level of worry, tension, restlessness and any panic symptoms.

Initial management

There may not be enough time to do everything in this first consultation. The following approach seems realistic.

1 Ensuring her safety until your next meeting is the priority. If there is a significant and immediate risk of self-harm or suicide the remainder of the consultation will need to address this. This may involve requesting crisis assessment by a community mental health team member or even admission to hospital for further monitoring of mental state, assessment and observation.

2 A brief plan to tackle any pressing problems. Discussing her problems may well have given her some relief. Helping her to devise a plan until the next meeting will help her to feel more in control. Success will bolster self-esteem and this is important. A problem-solving approach can be utilised.[9] This will involve: (1) identifying her main problems; (2) prioritising problems; (3) brainstorming/generating achievable solutions to immediate problem; (4) agreeing the solution to be tried.

3 Educational literature. If she fulfils the criteria for major depression provide some written material on depression. This should include details of possible treatment options. I regularly discuss how often people already feel out of control and disempowered by feeling like this and it is important that they feel fully involved in deciding how to manage it. Agree to discuss the options next time.

Subsequent action should include the following:

Investigate and treat any contributing biological factors

These might include thyroid disorder and menopausal issues.

Biological management

Exercise

A review of the evidence has led NICE (the UK's National Institute for Health and Clinical Excellence) to advise recommending structured exercise programmes consisting of up to three sessions per week lasting 45 minutes to one hour for mild depression.[10]

Medication

Medication counselling, including information about depression, has been shown to treble the odds of continuing with antidepressant treatment. Introduce the concept that the mind and body are not separate entities and that they influence each other: the chemical messengers of the brain are influenced by our thoughts and feelings (and vice versa). The depth of explanation will obviously be guided by her ability to understand (which will be influenced by the depression as well as her intelligence). I often tell the patient the following:

> 'Depressed mood is associated with a particular pattern within the brain chemical messenger system. Under normal circumstances the chemicals change as our moods change, depending on what we are doing/experiencing/thinking at the time. However, a situation can occur where the mood becomes "stuck down", no matter where you are, what you are doing, or who you are with. In this situation you do not get the same level of enjoyment out of activities. The chemical messenger system has become stuck in a depressed mood state and needs some assistance to correct its balance. We call this state "clinical depression" (or "major depression"). The problem is common. Whereas the average length of an untreated episode of clinical depression is eight months, we can use an antidepressant medication to help correct the chemical balance and "unstick" the mood. With this approach, positive changes often occur within two to four weeks.
>
> Antidepressants are not addictive. However, it is true that the brain gets used to their presence. For this reason, we stop antidepressants slowly so that the brain can adjust without difficulty.
>
> They take between 10 days and four weeks to start working.
>
> Their role is to "unstick the mood". Of course, the medication will not take

away problems but at least it will allow you some relief from the feelings of misery when you are distracted from your problems, for example when you [insert patient's hobby/interest].

You will be reviewed regularly so that any issues or concerns that you might have can be discussed.

Like all medicines, antidepressants can cause side-effects. The information leaflet that comes with the medication will describe many potential side-effects. These are not common and it is important to remember that any bad effects will stop when you stop taking the medication. It is possible that you will experience a degree of nausea and possibly a headache. These annoying effects will usually go away after 7–10 days.'

Which antidepressant should we prescribe? All antidepressants have a similar efficacy but there is a difference in tolerability; patients stop older tricyclic antidepressants (TCAs) (not lofepramine) more often than the selective serotonin reuptake inhibitors (SSRIs) and newer antidepressants because of side-effects. Studies show that TCAs are taken for a shorter time and less often at a therapeutic dose compared with the SSRIs. Patients frequently swap to SSRIs.

There will be the individual patient with individual factors to consider. She may have previous experience of medications. Establish what has worked before and use it again.

Some antidepressants bolster the transmission in one neurotransmitter system whereas other preparations are dual action. For instance, the SSRIs bolster the transmission of serotonin while mirtazapine and tricyclic antidepressants have both serotonergic and noradrenergic activity. It makes some sense to try someone on a dual action antidepressant if they have not benefited from single action.

Potential side-effects can be good or bad – some examples: night-time sedation might be helpful for someone whose sleep has been disrupted. Appetite stimulation from mirtazapine, for example, might be useful for someone who is also suffering cancer-related anorexia but not for someone who is overweight. Delayed ejaculation with the SSRIs might really boost the confidence of someone with a premature ejaculation problem.

Consider the potential for toxicity in overdose. It would be wise to avoid tricyclic antidepressants if there is a risk of suicide (with the exception of lofepramine).

Allow for concurrent illness and interactions. Avoid TCAs in ischaemic heart disease, prostatism and glaucoma. All antidepressant drugs lower seizure threshold although TCAs probably more so. St John's wort stops the combined oral contraceptive pill working and interacts with warfarin and possibly anticonvulsants. Citalopram or sertraline may be good choices for patients on multiple drug therapy as they have a lower potential for drug interactions. Take into account associated psychiatric disorder. When there is a strong obsessional component (*see* Chapter 8) a serotonergic antidepressant would be a better choice (e.g. SSRI).

Continuation treatment after treatment of the acute episode reduces the chance of relapse. The World Health Organization guidelines suggest six months of continuation treatment after the first episode. However, you will need to be guided by her attitude to taking medication and may need to compromise; feeling disempowered by taking medication will not help her depression!

Arrange to review her two to three weeks after commencing medication and regularly thereafter. Patients often gain more energy before their actual mood and negativity changes. This is important in someone who has been harbouring suicidal thoughts. They might not have had the drive to kill themselves before treatment. The initial stages of treatment, with increased energy, might heighten any suicide risk. Explain that there will not be a sudden improvement in mood; that there will be a few brighter moments breaking through the darkness and that these will get longer and more frequent; that it is the general trend that matters and not to panic if there are some bad days now and then.

The preparation and/or dose should be reviewed at six weeks if there has been no benefit.

Stopping antidepressants should be a gradual process over a few weeks. Guidance from NICE states four weeks, with some people needing longer. It can be helpful to test the water by reducing the dose every two weeks. For example, in the case of someone taking 20 mg citalopram daily, they could take 20 mg, 10 mg alternate days for two weeks. If they feel well, then they can reduce this to 10 mg daily for two weeks. If they still feel well they can reduce to 10 mg, 0 mg alternate days for two weeks then stop. Fluoxetine has such a long half life that it can be stopped more quickly.

Psychosocial management

Specific grief or relationship counselling may be useful in this case. If she lacks a confidant(e), non-directive counselling may be appropriate.

'Stepping yourself' into her situation (accurate empathy) is all important. She needs to feel as if we have been listening to her and understand her problems. Employ reflective listening – *see* Chapter 11 for more details. Additionally, there are psychological tools which can be successfully applied in your 10-minute consultation slots. Cognitive behaviour therapy has proven efficacy in the treatment of depression. Outlined below are some simple psychological techniques which are related to CBT.

Problem-solving approach as outlined earlier

This may reveal problems which require the assistance of outside agencies.

Self-help CBT

Discuss how thoughts, feelings and behaviours all affect each other; a change in one can bring about change in the others. Is she aware of how her thinking may have changed in her depression? Has it become more negative? Can she give an example? What was she doing when she thought like this? How did she feel when she thought like this?

She may benefit from self-help CBT:

➤ The MoodGym programme has proven benefit[11] and is available free at www.moodgym.anu.edu.au
➤ The CBT self-help manual – *Mind Over Mood* – by Dennis Greenberger, Christine Padesky (Guilford Publications; 1995).

Progress can be monitored at review appointments. Depending on available resources, a referral to a professional trained in CBT might be appropriate.

Find out how progress would be characterised in her individual case

1 Ask her to describe a period of time over the last week when things, although bad, were not quite as bad. Who was she with? (Does she like being with that person? . . . What is it about the person/setting that appeals to her? . . . etc) What was she doing? What was she thinking about? When she did that, how did she feel?
2 Ask her what she would expect to be doing if she were improving. How would that make her feel?

This approach often highlights the importance of socialisation and also helps to individualise the programme when it comes to goal setting.

Use the material obtained from this questioning as a foundation for improvement

Doing more of what works is important: certain people may bring more relief than others so can she spend more time with those people. Encourage her to do more of her progress-associated activities in a graded way. Setting realistic goals is important in promoting success (and therefore in building confidence and self-esteem).

Discuss 'vicious cycles'

When we are depressed we lose motivation and interest and as a consequence we do less. When we do less, we feel useless and are more likely to feel depressed and so the depressive cycle continues. She can break the cycle by two means:

1 waiting for the depression to get better. This approach is passive and disempowering and will not promote positive change
2 doing a bit more. If she plans her graded activity carefully and does not set her standards too high, then she is more likely to push through the 'motivation barrier' and succeed at something. This will in turn make her feel more effective and confident and will help her mood; feeling less depressed will help her to do more . . . etc . . .

If the low mood has been more long-standing or more entrenched the approaches set out in Chapter 13 might be helpful.

Psychotic depression

Hallucinations are more likely to be second person (talking at the patient) and mood-congruent; making derogatory comments about the patient; telling the patient to harm himself/herself.

Delusions are going to reflect the patient's negative view of himself/ herself, the world, the past and present. There might be the belief that they are fundamentally a bad person who has done bad things. They may suffer with nihilistic delusions. Nihilistic is the root of the word 'annihilate' and means destruction or death. People experiencing nihilistic delusions believe things like they are decomposing, their bodies don't work, their internal organs are rotten or solidifying or even that they are actually dead.

Psychotic depression will require treatment with an antipsychotic medication as well as an antidepressant by our specialist colleagues.

Depression in childhood and adolescence

Children and young people may not have reached a developmental stage where they are able to manifest all the recognised symptoms of depression; for example, ideas of unworthiness. Appetite and weight loss appear less often in children than in adults. It is therefore important to be alert to the possibility of a persistent and pervasive low mood as outlined above.

Referral for specialist assessment and advice should precede any prescribing of medications. The UK Committee on Safety of Medicines has issued guidance stating that the SSRI fluoxetine is the only SSRI and the only antidepressant that can be used to treat depression in people younger than 18 years.

Seasonal affective disorder – winter depression

The details of this topic are taken from a very helpful review article by Eagles.[12]

Symptoms typically commence in autumn or winter, peak between December and February and remit during spring and summer, during which seasons up to a third of patients become hypomanic, usually to a mild degree.

The symptoms are often those outlined above though about three-quarters of patients experience a significant increase in 'hibernation-type' features such as increased duration of sleep, while perceiving their sleep to be of poor quality. This is associated with daytime sleepiness, which often peaks in the late afternoon. A similar proportion of patients experience an increase in weight and in appetite, during which cravings for carbohydrate and chocolate are frequently prominent.

Light deprivation can be seen as the main cause of winter depression. There is also the 'phase-shift hypothesis' (as occurs in jetlag). The circadian rhythms of people with winter depression are seen as phase delayed with late onset of melatonin secretion, a pattern that can be corrected with morning light. Serotonin is also implicated. Various parameters of serotonergic function fluctuate seasonally and serotonin is linked intimately with the regulation of appetite and sleep.

Figure 7.1 illustrates how symptoms helpfully interact and improvement in one area positively impacts in other areas.

Discuss healthy eating strategies and recommend regular exercise routines

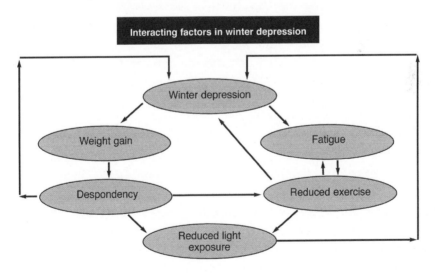

FIGURE 7.1 Features of winter depression

in the summer and to persevere with these to the best of their ability during the winter months. As much of the exercise as possible should be outdoors during daylight. If they can be afforded, sunny winter holidays (January may be the ideal month for many) are physiologically and psychologically beneficial. Social contact should be continued if possible, and in general it is helpful if friends and relatives know to anticipate, and attempt to tolerate, some degree of lethargy, low mood and irritability. The psychological approaches that have proven benefit for major depression should be just as applicable here. Reformulating negative thoughts is often helpful. For example, sufferers tend to focus gloomily on the relative certainty with which depressions recur, rather than on the knowledge that they will remit.

Light therapy

The stronger the typical winter symptoms are (such as hypersomnia, carbohydrate craving and weight gain), the more likely that light therapy will help and should be considered first choice. Bright light in the mornings is more helpful than bright light in the evenings.

If light therapy is to prove successful, response often commences within days and is usually apparent by the end of week one. If there has been no response in the first three weeks, then a subsequent response is unlikely. For this reason, it is appropriate that some lightbox suppliers have a sale or return policy within three weeks of initial purchase.

It is usually advisable, especially if patients are buying their own lightbox, to advocate that light therapy commences for the first time only once symptoms are clearly present; only then can effectiveness be assessed. However, in future winters, patients who respond to light therapy should usually start treatment as soon as the first symptom emerges. Light therapy prior to the onset of symptoms might prevent a winter episode of depression. Light therapy is usually phased out gradually in spring, often round about the time the clocks change, but this will depend on previous timing of symptom offset and current well-being.

Headaches and blurred vision are the most commonly reported adverse effects, occurring in up to 20% of patients. Feeling 'wired' (anxiously energetic as if after too much caffeine) is also fairly common. Rarely, hypomania may be precipitated. If used too late in the day, especially in people who are responders to light therapy, insomnia may well be induced. Light therapy might cause problems for patients on potentially photosensitising medication such as chlorpromazine, lithium or St John's wort.

Practical aspects of light therapy for winter depression

➤ It is most effective in the early morning.
➤ If it can be tolerated, users aim for a brightness of 10 000 lux. This equates to the eyes being 18 to 21 inches (45–53 cm) away from an average lightbox, and to start by using it for 30 minutes each morning.
➤ 30 minutes each morning is an appropriate initial duration of treatment.
➤ Responders usually improve within one week and not later than three weeks.
➤ Side-effects include headaches, blurred vision, insomnia and overactivity.
➤ There are alternatives to lightboxes, which include light visors and dawn simulating alarm clocks.

Antidepressants

Avoid sedative antidepressants; start with an SSRI. In patients with established winter recurrences, it is usual to instigate treatment as soon as symptoms re-emerge in the autumn and to phase out treatment in spring. For patients who also experience non-seasonal episodes, year-round prophylaxis may be deployed, sometimes regularly increasing the antidepressant dose during the winter months.

Postnatal depression

In the developed world suicide is now the main cause of maternal death in the first year post partum.

One of the consequences of our brains out-evolving our bodies is that we have forgotten our pack-animal needs. Many women who have moved away from their extended families for education and careers are left without the immediate practical and emotional support provided by the group. If a pack of supportive relatives were not needed, surely we would have evolved so that woman and baby hibernate for three months after parturition to allow adequate recuperation! A huge life event to adjust to along with possible issues of loss (loss of career, loss of the relationship to partner as it was), lack of sleep, hormonal influences (we know that oestrogen modulates the transmission of serotonin) might all contribute to a depressive vulnerability.

Being postnatally depressed is not just an issue for the suffering woman but can have consequences for the baby. The woman might become less emotionally available and this might impact on attachment. Research shows that postnatal depression can have an adverse effect on the cognitive, emotional and social development of the baby. Some good reasons then for identifying the problem and dealing with it!

The woman might not appear depressed – the term 'smiling depression' has often been used to describe postnatal depression. Underneath the smile could hide some worrying thoughts about whether life is worth living; feelings of guilt, inadequacy and despair. The woman might be having thoughts about harming the baby. These are often 'obsessional', i.e. unwanted thoughts coming into her mind and causing a great deal of distress.

The Edinburgh Postnatal Depression Scale (EPDS)[13] – see Appendix 2

One way of ensuring that questions about mood are asked routinely in a standard manner is to ask the mother to complete a questionnaire. The EPDS has been developed as a screening tool for the detection of postnatal depression, and validated for use, particularly at six to eight weeks postpartum. The EPDS is to be completed by the mother alone, at routine points of contact with health visitors.

Those scoring highly will be clinically assessed, by expanding on the questions and by exploring the context, the persistence and the severity of symptoms. Many women who score highly have a depressive illness. Some have mild, transient low mood. Some have other conditions such as anxiety disorder, physical illness, or social difficulties. Table 7.1 shows how to interpret the EPDS score.

TABLE 7.1 EPDS scores

1–8	9–13	14–19	20+
Normal	Possible depression	Probable depression	Severe disturbance

Management of postnatal depression

The following interventions may be considered.

➤ **Further regular review**: For mild or equivocal cases support and the passage of time may bring resolution, or clarify the need for further action.

➤ **Social support**: The challenges of motherhood can precipitate depression in women without supportive relationships or in adverse social circumstances. Improving these factors will help recovery. Support can be offered by primary care health professionals and by friends, relatives and any wider social network. A social worker may help to sort finances or housing applications. A health visitor or another mother can introduce a depressed mother to support groups. Relatives can be encouraged to give extra time and practical help.

➤ **Counselling**: Studies have found a favourable response to supportive psychotherapy at home for depressed new mothers. Non-directive counselling by health visitors has proven benefit.[14,15]

➤ **Antidepressants**: Consider when there is dysfunction, persistent and pervasive mood change and fulfilment of the criteria set out above. Ensure that the antidepressant prescribed does not have side-effects that hinder compliance and is suitable for breastfeeding mothers.

BOX 7.1 CASE STUDY – POSTNATAL LOW MOOD

I include this case as it illustrates how rich the experience of primary healthcare can be and how we benefit from that longitudinal relationship with patients and their families.

Mandy, my patient, aged 17 and with very little family support, became pregnant by Peter aged 18. Peter, also my patient, was raised by his grandparents after his mother died of cancer when he was aged six. On the day of the eight-week baby check I was surprised that Mandy did not attend with the baby. Peter came instead and told me he was worried about Mandy who was shouting a lot and not seeming herself. I had a chat with the health visitors and they later got back to me having spent some time with Mandy and getting her to complete the EPDS. Mandy had scored 13 and they were worried about her. Peter had seemed reluctant to allow Mandy to be seen alone with the health visitors; he had wanted to be with Mandy all the time. It was arranged for Mandy to come and see me. It became clear that her mood was not pervasively low. When she had the opportunity to see close friends she could engage in conversation and her mood would lift – she enjoyed their company to her usual level and looked forward to seeing her friends just as much as she used to. The main problem from her point of view was that Peter had become very possessive, not wanting her or the baby out of his sight. He was checking on the baby all the time. I arranged to see Peter. I had treated Peter before when he had developed strong obsessive thoughts about the possibility of having cancer. He recognised that the thoughts (after much reassurance) were not justified but the thoughts kept coming anyway and they caused a great deal of distress. The thoughts reduced in their severity and frequency with treatment using an SSRI. Before meeting Peter to discuss possible problems between him and Mandy, I had wondered if his obsessional thoughts might have generalised somewhat; that perhaps he had developed obsessive thoughts about Mandy and the baby. When he came he admitted to feeling tense all the time and having difficulty relaxing. He had recurrent thoughts that something was wrong with the baby and that something bad was going to happen to Mandy or the child. This had led him to follow her; to check on her whereabouts. Mandy was understandably finding his behaviour intrusive and this was the source of the conflict between them. It is possible that his experience of losing his mother was predisposing him to this over-concern about Mandy and the baby. His thoughts were obsessional in nature and he agreed to restart the SSRI. We discussed how his obsessional tendency was likely to be with him into the long term and may wax and wane depending on how much strain he was under. As his mental state improved, the relationship improved as did Mandy's EPDS scores.

In this case the EPDS indicated that further assessment was required. She was not clinically depressed though was at risk of developing clinical depression with the strain she was under.

We discuss obsessional thoughts in the next chapter.

ELEVATED MOOD

Just as mood can be persistently low to the extent that it causes distress/or dysfunction, it can also become persistently elevated. People can suffer from a single episode of mood elevation (hypomania or mania depending on severity) or can have recurrent episodes. Recurrent episodes can be interspersed with depressive episodes. When there has been greater than one episode of mood disorder with at least one being an episode of elevated mood, the condition is termed biploar affective disorder.

So there has to be mood elevation or irritability to a degree that is abnormal for the individual. Other features include increased activity, increased talkativeness, difficulty in concentrating, decreased need for sleep, increased sexual energy, reckless behaviour such as overspending, increased sociability or overfamiliarity. Mania rather than hypomania exists where there is severe interference with personal functioning. The increased talkativeness becomes a 'pressure of speech'; there is difficulty keeping to topic with a 'flight of ideas'; behaviour is inappropriate to the circumstances; there can be a grandiose content to thought. When mania is psychotic there are usually mood-congruent hallucinations/delusions.

Screening for mania

'Has there ever been a period of at least four days when you were so happy or excited that you got into trouble, or your family or friends worried about it?'
'Have you felt particularly cheerful and on top of the world, without any reason? . . . Too cheerful to be healthy?'
'How long does it last?'
'Have you felt particularly full of energy lately, or full of exciting ideas?'
'Do things seem to go too slowly for you?'

'Do you need less sleep than usual?'

'Do you find yourself extremely active but not getting tired?'

'Have you developed new interests recently?'

'Have you seemed superefficient at work, or as if you had special powers or talents quite out of the ordinary?'

'Have you felt especially healthy?'

'Have you been buying any interesting things recently?'

'Is there anything special about you?'

'Do you have special abilities or powers?'

'Is there a special purpose or mission to your life?'

'Are you especially clever or inventive? How do you explain this?'

'Are you a prominent person or related to someone prominent, like royalty?'

Remember the diagnostic hierarchy

Could this be a frontal lobe tumour? A tumour might present with symptoms of raised intracranial pressure – headaches worse first thing in the morning that might wake the patient, nausea, drowsiness. There may be other neurological symptoms and signs.

Could this be an amphetamine psychosis? Take a drug history and consider sending a urine sample to the lab for a drugs screen.

Seek early specialist help

Pathologically elevated mood can put the patient at risk so enlist the help of a specialist team.

REFERENCES

1. Whooley MA, Avins AL, Miranda J, *et al*. Case finding instruments for depression: two questions as good as many. *J Gen Intern Med*. 1997; **12**: 439–45.
2. Arroll B, Khin N, Kerse N. Screening for depression in primary care with two verbally asked questions: cross sectional study. *BMJ*. 2003: **327**: 1144–6.
3. American Psychiatric Association. *Diagnostic and Statistical Manual of Mental Disorders (DSM-IV)*. 1994.
4. Holleyman JA, *et al*. Double-blind placebo-controlled trial of amitriptyline among depressed patients in general practice. *BJGP*. 1988; **38**: 393–7.
5. Elkin I, Shea MT, Watkins JT, *et al*. National Institute of Mental Health Treatment of Depression Collaborative Research Program. General effectiveness of treatments. *Arch Gen Psychiatry*. 1989; **46**(11): 971–82.
6. Dunlop SR, Dornseif BE, Wernicke JF, *et al*. Pattern analysis shows beneficial effect of fluoxetine treatment in mild depression. *Psychopharmacol Bull*. 1990; **26**: 173–80.
7. Lima MS, Moncrieff J. A comparison of drugs versus placebo for the treatment

of dysthymia: a systematic review. *The Cochrane Library*. Cochrane Collaboration. Oxford: Update software; 1998.

8. Williams JW, Barrett J, Oxman T, *et al*. Treatment of dysthymia and minor depression in primary care: a randomized controlled trial in older adults. *JAMA*. 2000; **284**: 1519–26.

9. Mynors-Wallis LM, *et al*. Randomised controlled trial comparing problem solving treatment with amitriptyline and placebo for major depression in primary care. *BMJ*. 1995; **310**: 441–5.

10. www.nice.org.uk

11. Christensen H, Griffiths KM, Jorm AF. Delivering interventions for depression by using the internet: randomised controlled trial. *BMJ*. 2004; **328**: 265–8.

12. Eagles JM. Light therapy and the management of winter depression. *Advances in Psychiatric Treatment*. 2004; **10**: 233–40.

13. Cox JL, Holden JM, Sagovsky R. Detection of postnatal depression: development of the 10-item Edinburgh postnatal depression scale. *Br J Psychiatry*. 1987; **150**: 782–6.

14. Holden JM, Sagovsky R, Cox JL. Counselling in a general practice setting: controlled study of health visitor intervention in treatment of postnatal depression. *BMJ*. 1989; **298**: 223–6.

15. Ray KL, Hodnett ED. Caregiver support for postpartum depression. *Cochrane Database Syst Rev*. 2001; (3): CD000946.

CHAPTER 8

Anxiety-related problems and medically unexplained symptoms

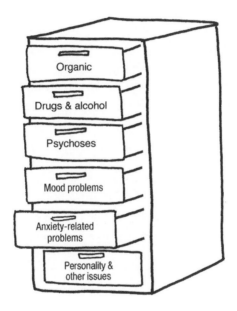

Anxiety is an unpleasant state of fearfulness with unwanted and distressing physical symptoms.

It is a normal response to a perception of a threat or danger (for example, spotting a lion while mowing the lawn!) and is biologically associated with the more primitive parts of the brain and the 'fight or flight' response. Referring to Part Four, Patient resources – anxiety biology reminds us of the cascade of events that occur in the anxiety response and the symptoms that are frequently experienced.

REMEMBER THE DIAGNOSTIC HIERARCHY

➤ Thyrotoxicosis.
➤ Excessive caffeine or recreational drugs (stimulants) – common.
➤ Phaeochromocytoma – rare.
➤ Accompanying depression or other diagnosis from the hierarchy.

WHEN IS IT A PROBLEM?

Anxiety becomes a problem when:
➤ we get into a habit of over-exaggerating danger
➤ we psycho-biologically get stuck in 'overdrive' – *see* Chapter 2, 'Biology' – if you need reminding of what I mean by this.

In these two situations we experience anxiety inappropriately. We might be worrying to an extent that is not completely justified. We might start experiencing panic symptoms out of the blue in the absence of a threat. We might become persistently tense and restless and have difficulty relaxing.

So it seems a state can develop whereby there are inappropriate, stuck neural and hormonal anxiety messages being released into the system. Treatment can aim to stop these inappropriate messages or to stop the body's response to them.

All anxiety problems tend to have a long-term course, with worsening at times of stress. The 'gut ulcer' analogy can be helpful when discussing this with patients. Gut ulcers can be calmed down with medications and lifestyle changes but can be prone to flaring up from time to time.

CATEGORIES OF ANXIETY

Ask yourself:

> 'Is it there all the time or does it come and go?' If it comes and goes, is it a response to a situation. Is the situation external or internal (distressing thought).'

All the time ('free-floating') = generalised anxiety disorder

> 'Have you been worrying a lot?'
> 'Do you feel tense?'
> 'Can you relax?'

Comes and goes (episodic) – *see* Figure 8.1 below

In the real world, problem areas frequently overlap. People often suffer both generalised anxiety and panic symptoms. Phobic problems often present themselves with generalised anxiety problems.

Before we focus in more depth on the specific types of anxiety and their management, it will be helpful to consider general anxiety management advice that can be applied across all diagnoses.

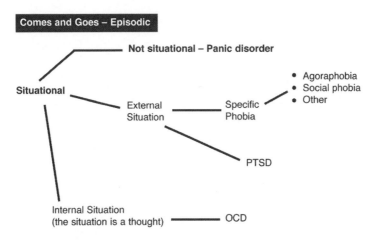

FIGURE 8.1 Types of episodic anxiety

GENERAL PRINCIPLES FOR PSYCHOLOGICAL MANAGEMENT OF ANXIETY PROBLEMS

These can be used in all specific anxiety problems.

Instruction on how to breathe to help physical symptoms

Breathe in for three seconds and out for three seconds and pause for three seconds before breathing in again.

Use before and during situations that make you anxious.

Regularly check and slow down breathing throughout the day.

Daily relaxation exercises such as meditation techniques can help to retrain the system stuck in overdrive. Practising for 10 minutes in the morning or at night can really help. Staying with breathing, the following technique can easily be taught:

> Choose a quiet place and time and either sit or lie down. Close the eyes. Place a hand on your abdomen. Become aware of your breath.

Allow the air to flow in and out through the nose at a depth and pace that you would use if smelling a lovely scent (such as the scent of a rose).

Breathe in with that steady breath for three seconds and then breathe out for three seconds and, if you like, hold the breathing for three seconds before breathing in again. When you breathe in your hand should rise and then fall with the out breath.

The exercise can be further enhanced by mentally focusing on the inner point between the breathe in and breathe out, and focusing on the outer point between the breathe out and the breathe in. If the mind wanders, do not become frustrated; just bring the attention back to the breath. With daily practice it becomes easier to reach a pleasant state of relaxation.

Dealing with worrying thoughts – challenging negative thoughts

Looking at whether extreme negative thoughts are fully justified. Negative thoughts associated with anxiety often centre around the possibility of future misfortune.

The self-help CBT resources listed in the previous chapter can help with this.

Dealing with worrying thoughts – distraction from worrying thoughts

There might be worrying thoughts about the anxiety symptoms (e.g. 'I am going to die' when one notices palpitations during a panic attack) or there might be worrying thoughts that are triggering the anxiety (e.g. 'what if the plane crashes?').

Examples of distraction techniques:

➤ Mental games such as singing a song, reciting a poem.
➤ Focusing attention on something associated with happy, relaxed experiences.
➤ A physical activity such as washing up or handing out drinks.
➤ Talking to someone.

Discuss lifestyle modification to manage stress and demands

Take account of those external features that are associated with endangering our well-being.

Where possible aim to reduce exposure to events that are perceived as being:

➤ uncontrollable
➤ unpredictable
➤ a challenge to one's capabilities and self-concept (because, in the short term our self-concept cannot be easily changed).

Reduce unacceptable uncertainties in one's situation

Figure 8.2 revisits the stress-performance curve from Chapter 2. When the demand is increased beyond a critical point there is a danger of attempting to do too much, too well and in too short a space of time. Getting the 'Human Doing-Human Being' balance is important.

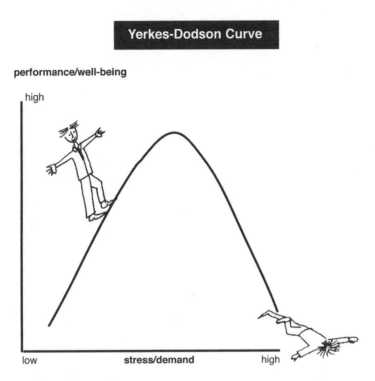

FIGURE 8.2 Yerkes-Dodson Curve

Avoid avoiding

Avoiding an anxiety-provoking situation will perpetuate the anxiety. Face the situation in a gradual step-by-step fashion. Anxiety levels will go up but if one remains in the situation, the anxiety levels will diminish again. Couple this graded exposure with breathing as above.

GENERALISED ANXIETY DISORDER (GAD)

Here there is pervasive, severe worry or anxiety about several different things.

There may be any of the symptoms described in Part Four, Patient resources – anxiety biology. Commonly experienced are restlessness, feeling tired easily, poor concentration, irritability, muscle tension and poor sleep. Sometimes these symptoms are more obvious to the patient than any problematic worrying thoughts.

The CBT approaches above can be very helpful in stopping the inappropriate anxiety messages. The SSRI, SNRI antidepressants are also effective at stopping them. Beta-blockers such as propranolol can be helpful in calming the body's response to the anxiety messages (the sympathetic nervous system 'fight-or-flight' response) though there is little available evidence to support their use. The calming effect of benzodiazepines should be reserved for short-term (one to two weeks) use in the case of extreme anxiety because of their addictive potential. In extreme anxiety they can be used alongside an antidepressant to give some relief while the antidepressant takes effect (can be two weeks or so – sometimes earlier, sometimes later).

PANIC DISORDER

Here there is a sudden onset of severe anxiety that may last only minutes or up to an hour. This anxiety is not situational; it arises 'out of the blue'.

Commonly people experience a feeling of not getting enough breath into their lungs, choking, butterflies, dizziness, sweating, palpitations and trembling.

A vicious cycle can develop as shown in Figure 8.3 below.

The importance of using the breathing technique during an episode should be emphasised. This really can help to control symptoms. The SSRI anti-depressants can help to switch off those stuck brain messages. CBT can help to challenge the thoughts that perpetuate a panic (e.g. 'I'm going to die').

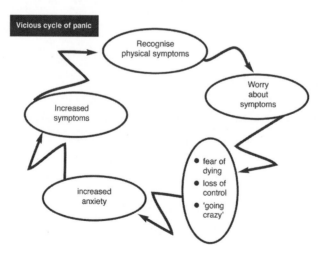

FIGURE 8.3 Vicious cycle of panic

SPECIFIC PHOBIAS (FEAR OF A PARTICULAR OBJECT OR SITUATION)

Phobias can develop as a conditioned response.

Examples of specific phobias

➤ Agoraphobia (with or without panic) – unreasonably strong fear of people, specific places or events.
➤ Social phobia – fear of social situations; fear of being criticised, scrutinised.

Psychological treatment of specific phobias

➤ Avoiding avoidance.
➤ Exposure therapy
  – Exposure to the anxiety provoking situation in a graded way while using relaxation (e.g. breathing) techniques and cognitive techniques to deal with problem thinking. An example in the case of social phobia:
    1   easy stage – walking with friend
    2   moderate stage – lunch with friend
    3   hard stage – shopping alone.

There may need to be a number of smaller steps along the way. It is important to remain at each stage until anxiety decreases to an acceptable level. When planning an exposure programme it can be worth considering 'exceptions' – for example: 'Can you tell me about the times over the last few months when, although it has been uncomfortable to mix with people, you have managed to do it?' – elaborate as outlined in Chapter 13, Psychological tools for general use. This will help to establish what is already working: a foundation on which to build.

Beta-blockers may be helpful as an adjunct to psychological treatment.

OBSESSIVE-COMPULSIVE DISORDER (OCD)

Here there are distressing recurrent and persistent thoughts or acts which the person recognises as their own, but has no apparent control. Thoughts keep coming despite their unwanted nature.

The recurrent thoughts are called obsessive thoughts. They may concern contaminating oneself or others, harming others, going against a social taboo. These thoughts are often accompanied by compulsions/rituals which are acts carried out time and again to reduce anxiety even though the person knows that they are silly and tries to resist them.

Screening for OCD

➤ 'Do you wash or clean a lot?'
➤ 'Do you check things a lot?'
➤ 'Is there any thought that keeps bothering you that you would like to get rid of but can't?'
➤ 'Do your daily activities take a long time to finish?'
➤ 'Are you concerned about orderliness or symmetry?'
➤ 'Do these problems trouble you?'

Using a 'vinyl analogy', there is a broken record type situation going on with the same mental experiences being played over and over again. Functional brain scan imaging can identify the biological home of this unhelpful situation. Cingulate gyrus and caudate nucleus circuits are involved with increased metabolic activity in the basal ganglia. Research has shown that these biological changes can be reversed by cognitive behavioural approaches to the problem. The concept of there being stuck 'false brain messages' can be helpful to patients: 'I feel the need to wash my hands again' becomes 'That nasty compulsive urge – false brain message – is bothering me again'.

Psychological aspects for discussion with the patient

Responsibility issues

The patient might benefit from considering the significance of the concept of responsibility in their life – do they have an exaggerated sense of responsibility? Table 8.1 illustrates the relationship between beliefs concerning self-responsibility and mental health issues.

TABLE 8.1 Responsibility issues

Attitude	Past catastrophe	Future catastrophe
High responsibility	Guilt, low self-esteem, depression	OCD
Low responsibility	Resentment	Anxiety, phobia

Exposure and response prevention

Exposure as per phobia and response prevention by managing anxiety and resisting compulsive behaviour.

Avoid avoiding intrusive thoughts – the more you try to push them out of the way, the stronger they can bounce back. Deliberately think about the thought for 10 minutes each day. Set limits on compulsive behaviour.

➤ 'A thoughtie is not a naughty'!
➤ 'Repeat your fears until bored to tears.'
➤ 'I must refrain to untrain my brain.'[1]

Medication

The SSRIs fluoxetine, paroxetine and sertraline are licensed to treat OCD.

SSRIs are often needed at higher doses and for longer to achieve an adequate effect.

As there is no evidence of differing efficacy, choice is dependent on side-effect profile. Gradually increase dose to the maximum within six to eight weeks of treatment initiation. An adequate trial is 12 weeks at maximum tolerated dose. Treat for at least 12 months. Discontinuation should be gradual. Clomipramine may also be effective.

Obsessive-compulsive spectrum

There are plenty of mental health problems which involve recurrent mental events. These can be considered to be part of an obsessive-compulsive spectrum. People with hypochondriasis have recurrent thoughts about the possibility of having something the matter physically. Other people experience a recurrent need to self-harm, binge or gamble. It has been theorised that the obsessive-compulsive spectrum can be split in two:

1 impulse control disorders – maximising pleasure, arousal and gratification. Self-harm, sex and gambling compulsions, risk seeking. It has been postulated that there is low level presynaptic serotonin in the frontal lobes and that SSRI medication can bring about a swift response

2 compulsive – avoid harm. The individual reduces anxiety with rituals – high presynaptic serotonin in frontal lobes and SSRI medication takes longer to impact on symptoms.

POST TRAUMATIC STRESS DISORDER (PTSD)

This is a prolonged/delayed response to an exceptionally stressful event in which the person was at risk of death or serious injury, or witnessed it in others.

Features include:

➤ *Nightmares, flashbacks* –'Have you had nightmares about it or thought about it when you did not want to?'

There's lots of evidence of structural changes to the hippocampus in people with chronic flashbacks.

➤ *Numbness, detachment* – 'Have you felt numb or detached from others, activities, or your surroundings?'

➤ *Hypervigilance* – 'Are you constantly on guard, watchful, or easily startled?'

Activation of the amygdala and the hypothalamus-pituitary-adrenal axis is associated with hypervigilance.

➤ *Avoidance behaviour* – 'Have you tried hard not to think about it or went out of your way to avoid situations that reminded you of it?'

After a traumatic event the individual needs support. It is important not to jump into diagnosing PTSD but to encourage the person to utilise social support from family and friends or from other agencies such as Victim Support (www.victimsupport.org) in the UK. Debriefing soon after the event can worsen the outcome. One study showed that debriefing involving a review of the traumatic experience, encouragement of emotional expression, promotion of cognitive processing of the experience, giving of advice about common emotional reactions and the value of talking about the experience was associated with a worse outcome.[2] One possible reason for this is that early interventions may disturb natural psychological 'defences' against fear and distress.

Continue to monitor the mental state over four to six weeks and see how the emotional dust settles or otherwise. In the first four weeks if symptoms are causing distress or dysfunction, the person can be said to have acute stress disorder. If things are not really improving at four to six weeks, referral for CBT would be appropriate. CBT treatment should involve graded exposure coupled with relaxation and cognitive restructuring ('I'm vulnerable and weak' becomes 'I'm competent').

It has been theorised that the stress of extreme traumatic events can prevent the laying down of memories and it is because of this that people experience flashbacks of the traumatic event. The use of a technique known as Eye Movement Desensitisation and Reprocessing (EMDR) has been gaining popularity. It has been claimed that EMDR can help to lay disturbing memories to rest. It is believed that 'cross-hemispheric' brain functioning is necessary to process such memories as occurs during the Rapid Eye Movement (REM) stage of sleep. EMDR aims to replicate this. The patient mentally relives the experience and reprocesses it while following the practitioner's finger with his eyes. However, there is doubt about whether eye movements are essential[3] and some practitioners use other techniques to stimulate cross-hemispheric functioning such as finger tapping. Some studies have tried to determine which specific components of the intervention are necessary to achieve therapeutic effect and suggest that the evidence only really supports the desensitisation component – the graded exposure of the individual to stimuli associated with the trauma.[4]

For UK ex-service men and women who suffer from psychiatric disabilities, including post traumatic stress disorder, consider contacting the Ex-Services

Mental Welfare Society (Combat Stress) at www.combatstress.org.uk.
SSRI medication or venlafaxine can be used.

MEDICALLY UNEXPLAINED SYMPTOMS

Dealing and coping with uncertainty is an important part of primary care work. This becomes easier if we have a relaxed attitude towards what we can expect ourselves to achieve in our work – aiming to help people manage their health issues rather than expecting ourselves to 'cure them'. It seems that people actually believe we frequently cure medical problems! – Quite often, of course, we are just modifying or suppressing them to more comfortable levels. Think about it; how often do you actually cure something? And if you are someone who actually thinks you do this frequently . . . ask yourself whether you really dealt with the root or source of the problem. Most of the time, we have to admit to not knowing what the deeper cause of problems are – what switches the body into a state where it is attacking itself in autoimmune problems such as rheumatoid arthritis and other connective tissue disorders; what causes cells to divide in an uncontrolled manner and become cancerous. There is an element of mystery about it. This is OK. We also come to realise that a large number of presenting problems we simply cannot diagnose. We can exclude any serious pathology and then use 'time as a tool'. Many of these undiagnosed problems then just get better. So an acceptance of the limitations of our medicine is helpful.

Classification

Somatoform disorder

It can all seem a bit burdensome when a patient repeatedly presents with physical symptoms and requests for medical investigations, despite repeated negative findings and reassurances by doctors that the symptoms have no physical basis. This is a description of somatoform disorders. If any physical disorders are present, they do not explain the nature and extent of the symptoms or the distress and preoccupation of the patient. **Somatisation disorder** is a form of this state of affairs where the main features are multiple, recurrent and frequently changing physical symptoms. In **hypochondriacal disorder** the essential feature is a persistent preoccupation with the possibility of having one or more serious and progressive physical disorders. The level to which patients accept and believe reassurance varies. Occasionally the patient understands and believes the reassurances given but despite this has recurrent intrusive thoughts about the possibility of having a certain condition. You can see that this situation would fit on the obsessive-compulsive spectrum – see above.

Dissociative (conversion) disorder

This less common presentation used to be termed 'conversion hysteria'. It is presumed to be psychogenic in origin, being associated closely in time with traumatic events, insoluble and intolerable problems, or disturbed relationships. The symptoms may develop in close relationship to psychological stress, and often appear suddenly. The theory here is that certain emotional material is too painful to cope with consciously so it is repressed into the unconscious; it manifests itself by conversion into physical symptoms. Anna O was the pseudonym used for Bertha Pappenheim by physician and physiologist Josef Breuer in his book *Studies on Hysteria*,[*][5] written in collaboration with Sigmund Freud. She suffered from epilepsy; one of her arms was paralysed as a result of complex seizures. After study, it was discovered this was the arm she had cradled her dying father with. It was theorised that she was unconsciously stopping the use of the arm as punishment because she blamed herself for her father's death.

Through analysis with Breuer, it was discovered that by talking about what had happened when the symptoms started, she would recover a repressed fact and then recover a bit. This is what Pappenheim called her 'talking cure'. Breuer called the act of recovery through this method catharsis. This case was the beginning of psychoanalysis, which would be later heavily developed by Freud.

It is worth bearing in mind that much of Freud's work is now viewed with scepticism, and it may be that patients Freud thought were hysterical may actually have suffered from organic illness. A number of studies have shown that for patients who have seen a neurologist, the rate of misdiagnosis at follow-up is between 5% and 10%,[6-9] though this level of misdiagnosis is similar in other neurological and psychiatric conditions.

There is little evidence-based treatment of conversion disorder.

When to consider somatoform disorder as a diagnostic possibility

➤ Vague or complicated illness story.
➤ Not responded as expected to treatment.
➤ If symptom patterns repeat themselves in an incomprehensible manner.
➤ Where something does not really add up.

The approach

Fink *et al.*[10] developed The Extended Reattribution and Management Model for managing somatoform disorders. The spirit of communication described in the psychological tools chapters of this book will help to steer a more

---

* Originally published in Vienna in 1895 – *Studien über Hysterie.*

comfortable path in our journey with these patients. The journey will become shorter, with less unnecessary stopovers and the company will be more agreeable. I have adapted their work to complement the other content of this book and my experience as a general practitioner.

Make the patient feel heard and understood

One of the most important psychological aspects of the treatment programme is to: make the patient feel heard and understood. Using the **OARS** discussed in Chapter 12 will help.

O: **Open questions** – 'What . . . where . . . how . . . why . . .' etc. Closed questions lead to the doctor overcontrolling the conversation and a shift of responsibility towards the doctor (something that can feel an uncomfortable burden especially when there are no easy solutions or quick fixes!).

 We have to balance this with keeping focused. Typically such patients are vague about symptom description and elaborate greatly on how severe an impact symptoms are having on their lives. They often go off topic.

 If the patient spends too much time on irrelevant information, try to keep the focus by asking:
 ➤ 'It is fun to hear about the football match, but please tell me more about . . .'

A: **Affirmations**
 ➤ 'Yes, clearly this has been taking its toll on your relationship and it has been difficult for you to bring this today . . . how does . . .?'

R: **Reflective listening** – *see* exercise in Chapter 11.

S: **Summarising** – the following expressions can be used.
 ➤ 'Did I understand you correctly; you mean . . .,'
 ➤ 'If I have understood you correctly, you are saying . . .'

Working like this will reduce patient resistance to accepting and adjusting to the idea that there is nothing seriously wrong and that further investigations and treatment are unnecessary.

 Start with the history of the symptoms then use the same approach to:

Explore life events, stress, and other external factors
➤ 'What else is happening in your life (in general)?'
➤ 'How do you feel about this?'

➤ 'What causes you the most trouble?'
➤ 'How do you handle this?'
➤ 'How did you cope with this?'

Ask about depression and anxiety

➤ 'How is your general mood?'
➤ 'Are you able to relax?'

It is important to ask about psychosocial circumstances and relationships at the assessment stage rather than waiting until 'the final verdict' otherwise the patient may feel that you are trying to dismiss the symptoms as being 'all in the mind' because you cannot find anything else wrong. Giving equal weight to this psychosocial material now has the implication that it has equal importance in the causation and maintenance of the problem.

When I told the orthopaedic surgeon I once worked for that I was joining a psychiatric training rotation he announced that it was easy to diagnose someone who was 'mental':

> 'If I operate on someone and they don't get better then they are mental,' he said!

Putting his arrogance aside, he had a much polarised view of the human make up – biological and psychological. I suspect he wouldn't work well with somatising patients. We need to help our patients to accept that we are psychobiological in nature. They will often say that 'other doctors think it's all in my head' or that 'they think I'm making it up'. They have symptoms that are real and have a need to deal with them whatever the cause.

Somatisers may actually be biologically different. Research suggests that somatising patients lack a normal filter function, resulting in the patients being unable to ignore irrelevant stimuli. There have also been PET brain scan changes reported.

Be clear about the patient's Ideas, Concerns and Expectations (ICE)

If you are anything like me, you cannot read minds so remember to ask what the patient thinks might be going on, what they are worried about and what they think should be done and why.

Brief focused physical examination and indicated investigations

For example, listening to the heart sounds if the patient complains of 'heart trouble'. This reassures the patient that he or she is being taken seriously and that the physician is careful and meticulous:

'Nothing in your description makes me think that there may be something wrong with your heart. However, I would like to listen to it anyway.'

Be clear about the diagnosis (if you have one!) and that there is nothing medically serious or sinister going on

A patient is most likely to accept this if you show that you have an understanding of the condition they are worried about and have discussed the absence of related symptoms and signs. Never say that there is nothing wrong with the patient. You may, instead, use phrases such as:

'You are worried about having bowel cancer. Symptoms of this are change in bowel habit with persistent loose stools, blood mixed with the stool and unexplained weight loss, sometimes with abnormal lumps felt on examination of the abdomen. You have not lost any weight; have become a little more constipated rather than experiencing looser stools and have experienced no blood with the stool. Examining you, I can find no medical abnormalities. There are no abnormal masses and everything is behaving normally underneath my hand. I note that you had a colonoscopy two months ago – the test that detects any abnormal growths or cancer and this was entirely normal. You are feeling pain on the left side and this is often seen in bowel muscular tension, and it is completely harmless.'

Acknowledge the reality of the symptoms and communicate empathic understanding of the patient's emotional problems/statements

'I can see you are very troubled by your pains (symptoms). Fortunately, for your reassurance, I can tell you that nothing indicates a serious physical disease. Perhaps we could try together to look for other possible explanations for your pain.'

Discuss the limitations of medicine

Explain that a large number of the problems people bring to the surgery we are unable to diagnose. We can exclude serious pathology. Many of these undiagnosed problems then just get better. When the problem does not completely go away, it is possible to learn to manage them better.

Roll with resistance

You may find in the more severe cases that there is a long way to go before the patient can begin accepting that there is nothing seriously wrong. Maintain the empathic firm but friendly approach. How about this from Fink *et al*:[10]

➤ 'I can hear (or see) you are convinced you have heart trouble (or another organ). However, I can find no signs of changes of your heart, which is why we cannot offer surgical or medical treatment that will make the symptoms go away. On the other hand, there are several things you can do to feel better, which would also be the case if you did suffer from an actual heart condition. Would it be OK to take a closer look at these measures?'

Depending on the problem, one should discuss relevant possibilities; for example, see the following.

➤ 'It is a fact that exercise is important for your health condition; this also applies to people suffering from heart disease. How does this sound to you?'
➤ 'Many people are afraid that the heart may be harmed when exercising or that it may even kill you. Did you worry about this?' . . . 'I can reassure you that this is not the case. However, you will certainly feel worse if you do not exercise – try to keep busy, even though I do understand you may find it difficult.'

Address the mind-body link

Try to explain that tension or mental stress is commonly accompanied by physical symptoms and/or that it may worsen existing physical symptoms.

➤ 'All people might react with physical symptoms and trouble when having problems or feeling tense or stressed . . . it is harmless, but I do understand it worries you and it is unpleasant.'
➤ 'I often see such symptoms in stressed or tense persons; could this also be the problem in your case?'

Examples used to illustrate the point that the patient might relate include the following.

➤ The experiencing of palpitations, breathlessness, and other physical symptoms when frightened or nervous over something.
➤ Increased sensitivity to physical symptoms when depressed.
➤ The tightening of muscles when frightened or stressed. This can result in pains that may increase the tension and give more pain; resulting in a vicious circle.

Consider providing patient resources – anxiety biology when there is a strong anxiety component.

When the going is even tougher! – chronic, entrenched

More helpful suggestions from Fink *et al.*[10]

➤ 'Many people feel like you do. It is in no way a rare condition.' 'We have a name for it, somatisation.' (*The patient will in most cases ask what it is.*)

Explain that the fundamental cause is unknown, as is also the case for many other illnesses (e.g. essential hypertension). You could say:

➤ 'We do not know the actual cause or the mechanisms behind it, but it is subject to a lot of research' or 'We do know with great certainty that it is not caused by any hidden physical disease and neither traditional medical nor surgical treatment will help, but may actually worsen, the condition.'

State the likelihood of a biological basis for the disorder, which is supported by scientific evidence.

➤ 'Several studies indicate that the reason is changes in the brain and the nervous system and some people are more bodily sensitive than others. In other words, they do not filter physical sensations and symptoms as well as others and are therefore more troubled by the different symptoms.'

Assist the patient's understanding by using well-known examples such as when you think about fleas and lice, you start itching. The senses and your attention are sharpened. In somatising, the increase in attention is just much stronger. Furthermore, it could also be mentioned that it can run in the family.

Explain to the patient that how he or she acts and reacts to symptoms is important for his or her future well-being. The patient must learn how to cope with illness, that is, to function as well as possible in spite of the trouble he or she is experiencing and that it is important not to become physically unfit, which will just make things worse. It is also important for the patient to understand that he or she should not expose him or herself to unnecessary tests or treatments (i.e. accepting the limits of medicine), because this may harm the patient even more.

Future involvement for the chronic, entrenched

➤ Be proactive rather than reactive.
➤ Promote continuity; become the named practitioner for the patient and inform other medical colleagues.

➤ Book regular scheduled appointments – yes, that's right – actually arrange to see them again! This is an investment; you will see them less and save time in the long run . . . honest!

➤ Acknowledge the symptoms and their impact.

➤ Explore provoking and relieving factors; encourage more elaboration of relieving factors/influences and summarise with emphasis on what is working.

➤ Explore and encourage elaboration of how the patient is coping despite the symptoms.

➤ Broaden the agenda – *see* Chapter 13, 'Psychological tools – tools for general use'. Ask 'What needs to be different?' in order to begin exploration of preferred future and the thoughts, feelings and behaviours that would characterise this.

➤ Consider antidepressants – the SSRIs. There is evidence that these can be effective.

REFERENCES

1. Powell TJ. *The Mental Health Handbook.* 2nd ed. Speechmark Publishing Ltd; 2000.
2. Hobbs M, Mayou R, Harrison B, *et al.* A randomised controlled trial of psychological debriefing for victims of road traffic accidents. *BMJ.* 1996; 313: 1438–9.
3. Shapiro F, Maxfield L. In the blink of an eye. *The Psychologist.* 2002; 15: 120–4.
4. Cusack K, Spates CR. The cognitive dismantling of eye movement desensitization and reprocessing (EMDR) treatment of posttraumatic stress disorder (PTSD). *Journal of Anxiety Disorders.* 1999; 13: 87–99.
5. Freud S, Breuer J. *Studies in Hysteria.* 2nd ed. London: Penguin Classics; 2004.
6. Couprie W, Wijdicks EF, Rooijmans HG, *et al.* Outcome in conversion disorder: a follow-up study. *J Neurol Neurosurg Psychiatry.* 1995; 58: 750–2.
7. Mace CJ, Trimble MR. Ten-year prognosis of conversion disorder. *Br J Psychiatry.* 1996; 169: 282–8.
8. Crimlisk HL, Bhatia K, Cope H, *et al.* Slater revisited: 6-year follow-up study of patients with medically unexplained motor symptoms. *BMJ.* 1998; 316: 582–6.
9. Binzer M, Kullgren G. Motor conversion disorder: a prospective 2- to 5-year follow-up study. *Psychosomatics.* 1998; 39: 519–27.
10. Fink P, Rosendal M, Toft T. Assessment and treatment of functional disorders in general practice: the Extended Reattribution and Management Model – an advanced educational program for nonpsychiatric doctors. *Psychosomatics.* 2002; 43: 93–131.

CHAPTER 9

Personality issues

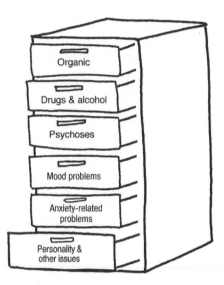

What are we dealing with in this chapter? Let us start by defining what is meant by **personality**.

> The distinctive and characteristic patterns of thoughts, feelings and behaviours that define an individual's personal style and influence his or her interactions with the environment.

We have discussed in the early part of this book the influence of genetics, parenting style and early environment on emotional development. Our early experiences shape our core beliefs about ourselves and the world. These core beliefs act as a mental filter that shapes our interpretation of events. We tend to extract information from our environment that is in keeping with core beliefs and pay little attention to anything that is not consistent with our core beliefs. Holding extremely negative core beliefs (e.g. 'I am unlovable') can therefore have profound consequences for our future relationships and well-being. We also explored Freud's personality structure (Ego, Id, Superego) and defence mechanisms which help understanding of personality dynamics.

In Chapter 11, 'Psychological tools – background considerations' we will be addressing transference issues. Transference is the projection of characteristics from a past relationship or a wished for/needed relationship onto a current relationship. In your working with patients with personality difficulties, be alert to transference issues.

The characteristics of our personality can protect us from or predispose us to the development of mental health problems.

There are a number of definitions available for **personality disorders** but I think the following will orientate us adequately:

Deeply ingrained, maladaptive patterns of behaviour, generally recognisable by adolescence or earlier and continuing throughout most of adult life, although becoming less obvious in middle or old age. Causes suffering to the individual or to others.

STATE (CATEGORICAL) VS. TRAIT (DIMENSIONAL) CLASSIFICATION OF PERSONALITY DISORDERS

Attempts have been made to describe distinct types of personality disorder (categorical classification) and these categories and their diagnostic criteria are to be found in the ICD-10[1] and DSM-IV diagnostic manuals.

Alternatively, there is the dimensional classification: the degree to which a person displays each of a number of personality traits and behavioural problems. In the real world, it is useful to have some knowledge of the various categories and their characteristics with an appreciation that the characteristics are on a spectrum of severity – and to consider using the term disorder only if these ingrained long-term characteristics are causing distress or dysfunction to the individual or distress to others.

In general practice, the patient may have been known since childhood and it can therefore be easier to distinguish an enduring pattern of behaviour from a new mental health episode.

SELF-ESTEEM ISSUES

Self-esteem: how worthy, lovable, valuable and capable we believe we are.

Low self-esteem is relevant to many of the personality problems that we are going to discuss. Low self-esteem is expressed in different ways.

There are three broad types of personality disorder: immature, mature and odd/eccentric. By giving an overview of the main issues I hope to aid our understanding of people with strong personality traits and therefore help us in our communication and relationships with them. Though we might not be seeing them with the aim of treating their personality problems, their personalities will colour how they present to us in their health-related consultations.

IMMATURE – DRAMATIC, EMOTIONAL, OR ERRATIC

These can be considered 'immature' personality traits with a hunger for attention.

There is the hope of maturation over many years with a mellowing of the traits.

Dissocial (psychopathic/sociopathic/antisocial)[1]

Disregard for social obligations, and callous unconcern for the feelings of others. There is gross disparity between behaviour and the prevailing social norms. Behaviour is not readily modifiable by adverse experience, including punishment. There is a low tolerance to frustration and a low threshold for discharge of aggression, including violence; there is a tendency to blame others or to offer plausible rationalisations for the behaviour bringing the patient into conflict with society.

Emotionally unstable (borderline)[1]

Definite tendency to act impulsively and without consideration of the consequences; the mood is unpredictable and capricious. There is a liability to outbursts of emotion and incapacity to control the behavioural explosions. There is a tendency to quarrelsome behaviour and to conflicts with others, especially when impulsive acts are thwarted or censored. Two types may be distinguished: the impulsive type, characterised predominantly by emotional instability and lack of impulse control, and the borderline type, characterised in addition by disturbances in self-image, aims and internal preferences, by chronic feelings of emptiness, by intense and unstable interpersonal relationships, and by a tendency to self-destructive behaviour, including suicide gestures and attempts.

Histrionic (hysterical)[1]

Shallow and labile affectivity, self-dramatisation, theatricality, exaggerated expression of emotions, suggestibility, egocentricity, self-indulgence, lack of consideration for others, easily hurt feelings, and continuous seeking for appreciation, excitement and attention.

Impulsive acts without consideration for consequences; behavioural explosions (tantrums when not getting own way!); efforts to avoid abandonment (often extreme behaviours or threats of suicide in order to influence others); affective instability (unstable immediate mood state – suddenly feeling very bleak/angry/anxious); suggestibility; theatrical – being the centre of attention (egocentric); attitude of irresponsibility – these are some of the immature 'toddler-like' characteristics. These characteristics not only bring distress/ dysfunction to the individual, but can also cause distress to others.

Psychological issues

We have learnt how attachment and parenting styles can influence future mental health in Chapter 1. The 'pickling' of young brains through the use of illicit drugs also prevents brain and personality maturation. These personality characteristics were associated with those people who took drugs 'to get by' in Chapter 5. In our relationships with these patients we really have to adopt an appropriate parenting role with the provision of a secure base and appropriate boundaries as discussed in the case example in Chapter 11.

We can find that people with strong emotionally unstable or histrionic traits are dominated by an urgent need to please others – there is a hunger for attention. Though they may seem to be attention seeking, on a deeper level they are attachment seeking. There is dramatisation and exaggeration, seductiveness – either social or overtly sexual in manner, immature and unrealistic dependence upon others. There might have been unstable attachment formation in early life and they may well have been disregarded in childhood; they are now looking in their current relationships for the attention they did not receive as a child – projecting that 'needed' aspect of their past neglectful relationships with parents – demanding total acceptance and protection and will seek it out with behaviour aimed at influencing others. Remember, it is OK to be manipulated, so long as you know you are being manipulated! The late psychiatrist and psychotherapist Anthony Storr wrote, 'It has often seemed to me that, if human beings have not been given what they need at the appropriate stage of their development, they are left with a compulsive hunger which drives them to try and obtain what has been missing'.[2] They may project their past experiences of authority figures (parents) onto us health professionals, seeing us as some form of authority – expecting us to disregard them and not take them seriously. As a consequence, they will be sensitive to anything that could mean we are being dismissive or uncaring (e.g. yawning during the consultation or having to change a consultation appointment for reasons out of our control). This misinterpretation may result in hostile behavioural/verbal explosions from time to time.

Simply removing the patient from your list and refusing to see them will just perpetuate the problem over time. We might find it difficult to cope with, this swinging from hot to cold – telling us we are the 'bee's knees' and then accusing us of not caring. We might become suspicious of their motives and prone to resentment. It is best if we can learn to control our immediate emotional response; to remain firm but friendly, to recognise the problem for what it is. Over time, the provision of this secure base is most likely to aid maturation – as the person learns that not all people are malevolent and are not going to desert them.

Use of the general psychological tools in Part Three will also help in the long-term management – as well as helping the patient, these tools can provide us with some protection during these emotionally demanding encounters. The approaches will help us to discover the strengths and resources that the patients have as well as learning that there is more to them than their problems!

The 'dissocial personality disorder' label has really stirred up some problems for the medical profession. In the UK the way the profession has communicated with the public over this issue as well as a difference in the understanding of the term 'disorder' between those working in the field and the general public has not helped. Take a look at the ICD-10 definition.

➤ Disregard for social obligations.
➤ Callous unconcern for the feelings of others.
➤ There is gross disparity between behaviour and the prevailing social norms.
➤ Behaviour is not readily modifiable by adverse experience, including punishment.
➤ There is a low tolerance to frustration and a low threshold for discharge of aggression, including violence.
➤ Tendency to blame others, or to offer plausible rationalisations for the behaviour bringing the patient into conflict with society.

There is debate over whether someone fulfilling such extreme criteria should be 'medicalised' into 'disorderhood'.

My concern is that the continued stigmatisation and discrimination of individuals suffering from mental illness is perpetuated by the placement of offending dissocial personalities under the 'mental disorder' heading. The continued use of the word 'disorder' by psychiatrists in connection with offending psychopaths generates confusion. Most members of the public believe 'disorder' means 'illness' or 'disease' (and rightly so as this is the definition given in many household dictionaries). To them it implies suffering and a need for medical treatment.

I performed an experiment when I was working in specialist psychiatry. I read aloud the characteristics of dissocial personality disorder as documented above to some 'non-medical' acquaintances. When asked to summarise how they would describe a person with these characteristics, they responded with such words as 'nasty person' or 'someone I would not want to meet'. They were later surprised to learn that these characteristics defined a mental 'disorder'. Although this experiment is far from being good science, it does illustrate how misunderstandings can result from using such terminology without providing further explanation.

The ICD-10 states that 'disorder' is not an exact term, but is used to imply the existence of a clinically recognisable set of symptoms or behaviour associated in most cases with distress . . . Social deviance or conflict alone, without personal dysfunction, should not be included in mental disorder as defined here. The diagnostic guidelines for specific personality disorders state: 'The disorder leads to considerable personal distress.' Yet social deviance and conflict are easily identifiable in these people whereas personal dysfunction and subjective distress are not and this is where dissocial personality disorder differs from other forms of personality difficulty.

In the absence of other psychopathology (or other medical conditions needing treatment), health services surely cannot have a role in dealing with individuals at the 'disordered' end of the dissocial spectrum; 'Gross and persistent attitude of irresponsibility and disregard for social norms, rules and obligations' and 'Marked proneness to blame others . . . for the behaviour that has brought the patient into conflict with society' are two ICD-10 characteristics of dissocial personality disorder. Although all mental and behavioural characteristics exist on a continuum of severity, the use of such words as 'gross' and 'marked' imply existence at the severe end of the continuum. It is therefore questionable whether such people could constructively engage with the mental health services. In any case, they believe they have no problem. They are comfortable with themselves.

At some level we can sympathise with such people when we consider that there may have been an absence of early attachments perhaps with extreme neglect. Unfortunately feeling sorry for them will not promote the development of a much needed attitude of responsibility – an essential prerequisite for change.

Immature brain

Slow wave EEG activity and 'positive spikes' in temporal lobes have led some academics to suggest there is a cortical brain immaturity or dysfunction in the temporal lobes and limbic system in people exhibiting immature personality traits. However, there is no magic 'brain maturation pill'. A firm, friendly and consistent approach with a degree of flexibility is most likely to aid maturation. The level of flexibility in the relationship will be determined by the degree of the patient's maturity and also by the situation over which the flexibility is needed/requested.

BOX 9.1 CASE STUDY

As a relatively new psychiatric trainee I was involved in the care of an emotionally unstable man who had been admitted to hospital following an overdose. We soon learned that he had not been clinically depressed (there was no pervasive or persistent lowering of mood) but was subject to rapid changes in his affect (immediate mood state) and had felt extreme sudden low mood and self-hate following an argument with his girlfriend. The overdose was impulsive and he had not really wanted to die; he was probably aiming to influence the girlfriend, to keep her close to him. In the early days on the ward, he made a number of behavioural gestures and outbursts in response to the restrictions imposed on him by inpatient care. However, we maintained a firm approach and drew up a contract of care outlining his and our responsibilities. He responded positively to this and became more calm and controlled. I was very keen not to prescribe sleeping tablets because of their addictive potential. I was aware of the learning theory that said that should I have given in to his requests for sleeping pills, his requesting behaviour would have been rewarded and perpetuated. There is a concept called variable rate conditioning that says that if a behaviour is rewarded at a variable rate (no pattern), then the behaviour will be strengthened the most (this is how gambling machines hook people so well) and my intention was therefore to never give in. The old, wise locum consultant criticised me for being so rigid and helped me to negotiate with the patient a set number of sleeping tablets to last a set number of days to help him to sleep at this 'difficult time of distress'. This level of flexibility had been helpful. The patient felt that he was being listened to and worked even more constructively with the team.

Self-soothing

People who have not had good nurturing as a child have not internalised any warm, cosy feelings and their ability to self-soothe when confronted with adverse life events is severely compromised. Also, as we have seen, patients who have not had warmth, closeness and hugs become adults who cannot get psychologically or physically close. Learning to self-soothe through attachment with a good object such as a pet can be helpful. It can also be learnt by techniques such as massage, aromatherapy, and a wide range of complementary therapies, which teach the patient to relate to their body in a non-destructive manner. Regular meditation can help the person to get in touch with and cultivate positive internal feelings. It can help the person to develop a sense that *they are not* their problems, their difficult thoughts or emotions and that there can be a distance between them and these mental experiences. When there is distance from them, there is a better chance of developing control over them.

Medication issues

While there is no magic potion, some medications can have a role in management. Of course we need to be mindful of the risk of overdose. It is also important that the patient does not think that because they are being offered a medication they must have a biological brain malfunction problem over which they have no responsibility. The SSRI antidepressants have been used to help with impulse control. Carbamazepine has also been used to help with affective instability and aggressive behaviour. However, at this time, supportive research evidence for the use of medication is lacking.

MATURE – ANXIOUS OR FEARFUL

'Mature' personality traits; change less likely to occur; stable characteristics over time – hunger for approval.

Anankastic (obsessional)[1]

Feelings of doubt, perfectionism, excessive conscientiousness, checking and preoccupation with details, stubbornness, caution and rigidity. There may be insistent and unwelcome thoughts or impulses that do not attain the severity of an obsessive-compulsive disorder.

Anxious (avoidant)[1]

Feelings of tension and apprehension, insecurity and inferiority. There is a continuous yearning to be liked and accepted, a hypersensitivity to rejection and criticism with restricted personal attachments, and a tendency to avoid certain activities by habitual exaggeration of the potential dangers or risks in everyday situations.

Dependent[1]

Pervasive passive reliance on other people to make one's major and minor life decisions, great fear of abandonment, feelings of helplessness and incompetence, passive compliance with the wishes of elders and others, and a weak response to the demands of daily life. Lack of vigour may show itself in the intellectual or emotional spheres; there is often a tendency to transfer responsibility to others.

Whereas people with the previous traits have felt disregarded, these people may well have been scrupulously regarded, weighed in the balance, and found wanting; their parents may have been critical and often emotionally distant (authoritarian parenting styles). They may be subject to chronic low mood.

They are concerned about what others think of them – there is a hunger for approval. There can be a need for repeated reassurance from others and successes. There is often a lack of assertiveness and an over-concern with pleasing people. They feel ineffective and unable to trust their own judgement. In time they might learn that effort can bring about success; passivity might be transformed into ceaseless effort – the need to achieve at the next big thing in order to give some sense of worth. Once achieved, instead of being able to feel satisfied they can experience depression as they relax into the conviction of their own ineffectiveness.

Unlike histrionic personalities who try to please in a manner designed to gain attention, these people are quieter in their efforts to gain approval. Their low self-esteem is expressed through a more 'head-down' approach. Not wanting to offend, be blamed and being so needy of approval – 'antennae' develop which tell the individual what might upset, or what might please the other people around him. Because there is a constant adaptation and manoeuvring to the emotional state of others the person often becomes uncertain of their own feelings. Being guided by the opinions of others, they risk having no opinions of their own.

This is a description of the severe end of the spectrum and one would hope that, for many people, alternative core beliefs will gradually develop to provide some balance. It will take time and helpful interpersonal contact for the individual to realise that they are fundamentally more important than the sum of their external achievements and that their self-worth is not dependent on such achievements.

The psychological tools that are outlined later will help to bolster self-esteem and reduce dependency; they focus on strengths and resources and help shift the locus of control towards the patient.

ODD OR ECCENTRIC
Paranoid[1]
Excessive sensitivity to setbacks, unforgiving of insults; suspicion and a tendency to distort experience by misconstruing the neutral or friendly actions of others as hostile or contemptuous; recurrent suspicions, without justification, regarding the sexual fidelity of the spouse or sexual partner; and a combative and tenacious sense of personal rights. There may be excessive self-importance, and there is often excessive self-reference.

Schizoid[1]

Withdrawal from affectional, social and other contacts with preference for fantasy, solitary activities, and introspection. There is a limited capacity to express feelings and to experience pleasure.

Flattening of affect and indifference to praise and criticism are contained within the diagnostic guidance of the ICD-10 relating to schizoid personality disorder. These characteristics have also been identified in children who later develop psychosis, as we discovered in Chapter 6. Perhaps they also lie on a schizophrenia spectrum where the addition of adequate stress has the potential of precipitating frank psychosis.

Once upon a time there was a schizotypal personality disorder but this is now considered to belong to the schizophrenia spectrum and is now called schizotypal disorder.

Other than the contribution made by genetics why else might people prefer to be alone and reluctant to allow anyone close to them? Storr[2] gives three possibilities.

1 Fear that any relationship will end and that they would therefore be worse off than if they had never got emotionally involved (fear based on actual experience of loss as a child).

2 Fear of being dominated or overborne by another person to the point of losing an identity of a separate person (deprived of having a sense of effectiveness and potency as a child; not being allowed to achieve in own right; treated as a 'doll' or an 'appendage' to the parent rather than a person with a separate existence).

3 Fear of exhausting the other person (e.g. when parents have experienced more exhaustion than pleasure when trying to enter the child's world – this might have happened if parents have been older).

We usually develop our self-esteem by mutually fulfilling relationships. It has been theorised that the schizoid individual must enter into a world of fantasy in order to generate their sense of self-worth and effectiveness.

REFERENCES

1. World Health Organization. *The ICD-10 Classification of Mental and Behavioural Disorders. Clinical Descriptions and Diagnostic Guidelines.* Geneva: WHO; 1992.
2. Storr A. *The Art of Psychotherapy.* Martin Secker & Warburg Ltd, jointly with William Heinemann Medical Books Ltd; 1979.

CHAPTER 10

Eating disorders

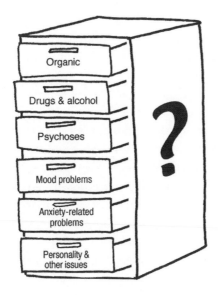

Where do eating disorders sit in our hierarchy?

There can be addiction, self-harm and obsessive-compulsive qualities to these problems. Beliefs about body image can sometimes seem delusional. When starvation occurs to the extreme, the biochemical ('organic') changes impact on cognition and mood.

We all know about the growing popularity of extreme diets. With about 5–10% of the adolescent girls in a GP practice using weight-reducing techniques other than dieting (vomiting, laxative or diuretic abuse, excessive exercising), body image and weight issues are an important issue. With numbers like these, we can assume that many patients presenting at a surgery will have background eating-disorder type issues and that some of these may develop into more serious eating disorders. Much of the hard fact and guidance in this chapter has been taken from the work of Janet Treasure of the Institute of Psychiatry, London.[1]

PRESENTATION

So how do we pick up these issues? Symptoms might include:

Physical

Loss of weight; amenorrhoea; other physical complications.

Psychological

Low mood; anxiety; irritability; obsessional symptoms, particularly related to food and weight.

Social

School or work problems; problems in the family and/or with relationships; arrests (usually for stealing) or other police contact.

ASSESSMENT

It is important to remember that the person may experience a lot of ambivalence about their problem and may find these issues extremely difficult to talk about. We need to question sensitively and the spirit of motivational interviewing needs to be applied in order to encourage engagement with assessment and management – see Chapter 12. Janet Treasure's team use the following metaphor:

> 'The sun and the wind were having a dispute as to who was the most powerful. They saw a man walking along and they challenged each other about which of them would be most successful at getting the man to remove his coat. The wind started first and blew up a huge gale; the coat flapped but the man only closed all his buttons and tightened up his belt. The sun tried next and shone brightly making the man sweat. He proceeded to take off his coat.'

The assessment may have to be carried out in several gentle chunks.

Where we suspect a problem in this area (and if we are good at remembering so many screening tools!) then we can use the SCOFF[2,3] – see Table 10.1. It has a sensitivity of 100% and specificity of 90% for anorexia nervosa. Although not diagnostic, two or more positive answers should prompt you to take a more detailed history.

TABLE 10.1 The SCOFF questionnaire

The SCOFF questionnaire
Do you ever make yourself Sick because you feel uncomfortably full?
Do you worry you have lost Control over how much you eat?
Have you recently lost more than One stone in a three-month period?
Do you believe yourself to be Fat when others say you are too thin?
Would you say that Food dominates your life?

What further questions might help establish whether this person has an eating disorder?

Obtain a description of eating during a typical day

What's eaten and when it's eaten.
➤ Whether there is any avoidance behaviour
 – avoidance of any type of food
 – avoidance of eating with other people.
➤ Is there any loss of control over the eating or any bingeing (eating a large quantity of food in a short space of time)?
➤ What sort of feelings arise during and after eating – what about guilt?

Do these feelings drive any other weight reducing behaviours?
➤ Vomiting.
➤ Excessive exercise.
➤ Abuse of laxatives and/or diuretics?

Background psychopathology?
➤ 'What do you think of your current weight? What do you see as your ideal weight?'
➤ 'How would you feel if you were the normal weight for your height?'
➤ 'How much of the day do you spend thinking of food and your weight?'
➤ 'Do you ever get depressed or guilty? Do you ever feel suicidal?'
➤ 'Has your life become more ritualised?'

Screen of important physical symptoms
➤ 'When was your last period?'
➤ 'Have you noticed any weakness in your muscles? What about climbing stairs or brushing your hair?'
➤ 'Are you more sensitive to the cold than others?'
➤ 'What is your sleep like?'

➤ 'Have you fainted or had dizzy spells?'
➤ 'Have you problems with your teeth (hot/cold sensitivity etc)?'
➤ 'Have you had any problems with your digestive system?'

Assess physical risk

TABLE 10.2 Physical risk

Measuring risk in people with eating disorders

	Examination	Moderate risk	High risk
Nutrition	Body mass index BMI = weight in kg/(height in m)^2	<15	<13
	Body mass index centile*	Below the third centile	Below the second centile
	Weight loss per week	>0.5 kg	>1.0 kg
	Purpuric rash	–	+
Circulation	Systolic blood pressure	<90 mm Hg	<80 mm Hg
	Diastolic blood pressure	<60 mm Hg	<50 mm Hg
	Postural drop	>10 mm Hg	>20 mm Hg
	Pulse rate	<50 beats per minute	<40 beats per minute
	Oxygen saturation	95	92
	Extremities		Dark blue/cold
Musculoskeletal (squat test**)	Unable to get up without using arms for balance	+	+
	Unable to get up without using arms as leverage		+
Core temperature		<35°C	<34.5°C
Investigations	Full blood count, urea and electrolytes (including PO$_4^{3-}$), liver function tests, glucose	Concern if outside normal limits	K$^+$ <2.5 Na$^+$ <130 PO$_4^{3-}$ <0.5
	Electrocardiogram		Prolonged QT interval (due to low potassium and magnesium)

*The body mass index centile plots body mass index against age. For adults a pragmatic classification system exists based on associations between body mass index and all cause mortality. The recently redefined body mass index categories are: underweight <18.5; ideal 18.5–24.9; pre-obese 25.0–29.9; obese class I 30.0–34.9; obese class II 35.0–39.9; and obese class III >40 kg/m². These fixed classifications are not appropriate for children, in whom the 50th centile for body mass index shows profound changes from birth through to early adulthood. Please refer to Centile BMI charts for children in Appendix 4.

**The squat test – a test for proximal myopathy: ask the patient to squat on their haunches and to get up without using their hands.

Disordered eating, often rooted in low self-esteem, can frequently be identified in primary care. Immediate, serious risks might exist and need to be addressed. More often though for the primary care practitioner, emerging, less well-defined presentations are encountered. Vicious cycles commonly exist and we might explore contributing factors. Situations that erode self-esteem will often fuel these problems. Asking about the times when, say, bingeing and vomiting have happened less often in the last few months might help to identify patterns of behaviour (what is happening, where it is happening and with whom it is happening) that bolster self-esteem and lessen the disordered eating. This sort of questioning is further explored in Chapter 13. It often helps with short-term planning.

BOX 10.1 CASE STUDY – ACHIEVING SOME SHORT-TERM EMOTIONAL RELIEF

Tara, who was losing control over her binge-eating, was in a negative spiral. While binge-eating, her feelings of emptiness and anger were momentarily soothed. However, she felt immediately guilty with self-hate and she would vomit up her food. She would then impose a strict dietary regime which was virtually impossible to abide by. Any minor transgression was interpreted as a severe failure and a need for soothing coupled with a severe 'sod it!' would lead to another binge.

We identified that there were some 'exceptions' – she fared better when she stayed at a friend's house for the occasional weekend. She would sleep better and related well to this particular friend. Feeling more respected and less tired led to a softening of her eating problems. She had been living in a shared house with noisy housemates who went to bed late. She had little in common with them. She was desperately in need of some improved control in the short term and we were able to discuss manipulation of her immediate environment, taking into account the helpful 'what, where and with who' factors that we had identified in our 'exception'.

Tara had appeared reasonably physically robust – we had some time to play with. The above took some of the heat out of the situation and we were then able to continue with our assessment of her problems along with intermediate/long-term planning.

CLASSIFICATION

Anorexia nervosa

1 Weight, measured as body mass index (BMI) < 17.5 kg/m² due to controlled eating.
2 Distorted body image and abnormal attitudes to food and weight.
3 Amenorrhoea and often other signs of starvation.
4 Thirty per cent of cases of anorexia nervosa have a chronic course. The morbidity and mortality of this group is considerable.
5 People with low self-esteem or who are perfectionists are more vulnerable.
6 Detecting the problem early in patients with unexplained weight loss improves prognosis.

Bulimia nervosa

1 Binge-eating real or perceived excessive amounts of food with loss of self-control.
2 Desire for thinness and preoccupation with food and weight.
3 Strategies aimed at weight reduction – vomiting, laxative and/or diuretic abuse, excessive exercising.

If there is also severe unexplained weight loss (body mass index <18 kg/m²) you should consider a diagnosis of anorexia nervosa of the 'binge-eating and purging' type.

Patients who have suffered with anorexia/bulimia nervosa for more than 20 years stand a 20% chance of dying from their illness, either by suicide or emaciation.

Binge-eating disorder

1 Binge-eating real or perceived excessive amounts of food with loss of self-control.
2 No use of extreme weight control strategies therefore often associated with obesity.

MANAGING EATING DISORDERS IN PRIMARY CARE

The approaches outlined in Part Three, Psychological tools will help with the development of a **therapeutic relationship** and exploration of the ambivalence surrounding behaviour change (*see* Chapter 12). Consider referral to a psychological practitioner to work on any relationship problems, perfectionism, rigid and anxious traits, sexual abuse, alcohol and/or drug abuse.

Offer expert information about eating disorders and their effects, and self-help resources. For those with internet access I recommend www.eatingresearch. com, the eating disorder information website from the Institute of Psychiatry. This provides a wealth of valuable information and useful links for the patient and those close to them.

Consider providing patient resources on disordered eating including the risks and self-help (in Part Four). This provides information about the health consequences of eating disorders as well as signposts to very good self-help resources.

MANAGING ANOREXIA NERVOSA IN PRIMARY CARE

When to refer

➤ You can manage patients with mild anorexia nervosa (body mass index >17 kg/m^2) and no significant comorbidities in primary care with support and monitoring. But if patients don't respond within eight weeks you should make a routine referral to specialist services.
➤ You should refer patients with moderate anorexia nervosa (body mass index 15–17 kg/m^2) and no significant comorbidities non-urgently to specialist services.
➤ Refer patients with severe anorexia nervosa (body mass index <15 kg/m^2), rapid weight loss, or evidence of system failure urgently to specialist services, or a medical unit if the physical status of the patient is life threatening.

If a patient is severely ill, particularly with medical complications or suicidal ideation, as described above, in-patient treatment may be needed to save a patient's life. Rarely the patient will have lost insight into the severity of the illness and will resist in-patient treatment. In these circumstances compulsory admission to hospital will be required.

Predicaments – family, patient and doctor

We are often confronted by a family who want us to 'do something' and to 'do it now' to stop the demise of their loved one. We might find ourselves in the middle of a professional conflict; on the one hand there is the obligation to act assertively if there are real immediate physical risks and on the other hand there is the knowledge that assertion, adoption of an 'expert' stance and appearing to want to rush change will just heighten resistance and threaten the working relationship and longer term change. . . . And the patient feels confronted by the family and confronted by that part of them that doesn't want to die and perhaps confronted by us because they fear we will lock them up and make them eat. She or he feels trapped; fearful of dying and fearful of putting on weight. So both we and the patient are caught in a difficult situation. I have found this common ground useful to discuss with the patient. The patient usually appreciates such honesty and occasionally we have even been able to laugh about 'the bloody mess' we both find ourselves in!

The natural need to help make their child better as quickly as possible can provoke/exacerbate over-involvement, criticism and perceived hostility – all of these are known to impair good mental health (*see* Chapter 1 – 'expressed emotion'). Acknowledge the predicament they are in. Educate the parents: anorexia is an illness and is not caused by stubbornness on the part of the patient. Parents need to be firm, consistent and empathic.

Nutrition and monitoring

➤ Weigh the patient regularly. The frequency of weighing and blood testing will depend on the rate of progress/deterioration.
➤ 'NICE's guidance (January 2004) recommends that in most patients with anorexia nervosa an average weekly weight gain of 0.5 kg in outpatient settings should be an aim of treatment. This requires about 3500 to 7000 extra calories a week.
➤ In the first phase (three to seven days) a soft diet is recommended of about 30–40 kcal/kg/day, spaced in small portions throughout the day. Oral supplements to help correct nutritional deficits such as Sanatogen Gold (non-NHS), Forceval 1–2, or Seravit capsules.
➤ Vomiting and diuretic and laxative abuse can cause severe dehydration (or over-hydration), acute renal failure, and electrolyte imbalance. Oral fluid and electrolyte replacement is preferable, for example with Dioralyte. Serum potassium levels may stay low despite potassium supplements if the patient continues to vomit.
➤ Be aware of the refeeding syndrome. In starvation the secretion of insulin is decreased in response to a reduced intake of carbohydrates. Instead fat and protein stores are broken down to produce energy. This results in an intracellular loss of electrolytes, in particular phosphate. When feeding begins, a sudden shift from fat to carbohydrate metabolism

occurs and secretion of insulin increases. This stimulates cellular uptake of phosphate, which can lead to a marked loss of circulating phosphate. This usually occurs within four days of starting to feed again and can produce clinical features which include rhabdomyolysis, leucocyte dysfunction, respiratory failure, cardiac failure, hypotension, arrhythmias, seizures, coma, and sudden death. Importantly, the early clinical features of refeeding syndrome are non-specific and may go unrecognised. Monitoring the physical state of the patient and blood biochemistry is very important.[4]

Medication

In anorexia nervosa, medication does not usually help associated symptoms of anxiety and/or depression. These will lift as the patient's weight improves.

MANAGING BULIMIA NERVOSA IN PRIMARY CARE

Aim to get them to eat three regular meals per day, which reduces the urge to binge.

Remember that there will be exceptions to the problem, times when it is less apparent. We can learn from these, as in the case of Tara outlined in Box 10.1. The self-help guides base themselves on cognitive behavioural principles with good evidence that many people can be helped by guided self-help using a book such as *Getting Better Bit(e) by Bit(e)* – *see* Part Four, Patient resources.

Description of cognitive behavioural strategies

In a 'food diary' table the patient is encouraged to document what she or he eats and when she eats it. She also documents how she was feeling before eating and what she was thinking at that time. She does the same for the thoughts and feelings that occurred after eating/bingeing.

The patient is then encouraged to see her behaviour and how she may change this – some examples are provided in the following.

➤ Decide that she will try not to vomit before 9am, and then 10am, etc.
➤ Decide on certain foods that feel 'safe' and eat those at times that feel more difficult.
➤ Plan to do something immediately after eating to take her mind off vomiting.
➤ Decide before she starts eating how much she is going to eat and try to stick to that.
➤ Only keep so much food in the house.

She is also asked to identify the negative thinking that fuels her negative feelings (using the diary), e.g. 'If I eat a chocolate bar, I will put on a stone', and underlying assumptions, e.g. 'all people who are fat are worthless'. She is helped to challenge such beliefs by discussion and support.

Medication
The SSRI antidepressants can be helpful in the short term.

NICE guidance
The UK's National Institute for Health and Clinical Excellence recommends that most adults with bulimia nervosa should have an evidence-based, self-help programme or a trial of an antidepressant as a possible first step, and 16 to 20 sessions of cognitive behaviour therapy over four to five months. You may need to modify the treatment for adolescents, according to their development and familial circumstances.

When to refer
Specialist referral is appropriate if:
➤ the patient doesn't make any progress
➤ there are strong concerns about physical or mental health
➤ you need to clarify the diagnosis or want advice about the best treatment
➤ you don't have access to evidence-based treatments, such as cognitive behaviour therapy.

REFERENCES
1. Treasure J. The Institute of Psychiatry. Available at: www.eatingresearch.com
2. Luck A, Morgan JF, Reid F, et al. The SCOFF questionnaire and clinical interview for eating disorders in general practice: comparative study. BMJ. 2002; **325**: 755–6.
3. Morgan JF, Reid F, Lacey JH. The SCOFF questionnaire: assessment of a new screening tool for eating disorders. BMJ. 1999; **319**: 1467–8.
4. Hearing SD. Refeeding syndrome is underdiagnosed and undertreated, but treatable. BMJ. 2004; **328**: 908–9.

PART THREE

Psychological tools

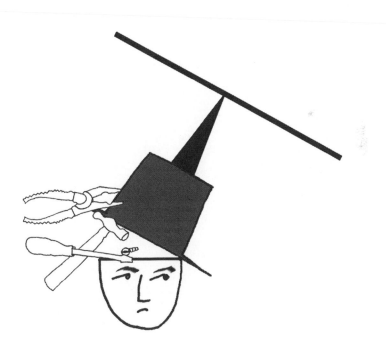

CHAPTER 11

Psychological tools: background considerations

BUILDING OUR CONFIDENCE

'I don't have the skills or time to help my patients psychologically.'

This thought is rather extreme and negative and the owners tell me it brings with it feelings of disempowerment and of a 'sinking heart' in some consultations. There is little evidence to support such a thought. In fact, there is more evidence to say that we can contribute towards positive psychological change and we don't need years of psychological training to achieve this. I hope that by the end of this part of the book you will agree with me at least in part. If you begin to develop a more balanced thought (cognition) regarding the value of your input such as:

'Well, actually, I already have some valuable skills and now I can build on them to make even more of a useful contribution'

then the construction of these chapters will have been worth it for me and the reading of the chapter will have provided some self-help cognitive therapy for you!

Before getting into specific approaches, let's consider some background issues and themes.

In primary care, there isn't time for long consultations. However, there can be frequent, short (10-minute) encounters. Only psychological interventions that lend themselves to 'chunking down' into smaller parts will be of any use.

There is also the issue of what can appropriately be applied given time restriction and skill level. In psychodynamic psychotherapy, expression of feelings and consideration of their significance along with the development of insight into the role of unconscious mechanisms is deemed to be important. It is postulated that painful memories and feelings are diverted or buried in the subconscious; that symptoms represent an emotional boil or abscess unable to find a path to the surface and that it is important to lance it to make therapeutic progress and bring psychological relief. The general practitioner cannot be expected to work at this deeper level but an awareness of transference issues (see below) and a very good understanding of the patient's background and circumstances can be put to good use. On top of this firm foundation, some simple approaches can be learned and applied. For those readers who are interested in learning more about the technique and theory of dynamic psychotherapy I recommend Malan's book which includes fascinating case studies.[1]

Research suggests that establishing a therapeutic alliance is key to bringing about positive change. The specific approach to therapy probably matters less than whether the person feels they can relate to you; whether they can get on with you. Using general practitioners as an example, there may already be a relationship with the patient that goes back years. This combined with the fact that the patient is here with their difficulty right now suggests that there is already a fair element of 'getting along with' going on.

Counselling, without additional factors such as practical help, mutual self-help or training in coping skills, has not been shown to produce sustained benefit, despite generally high user satisfaction. Therefore, becoming 'expert' counsellors is perhaps not what we should be striving for. Building on our relationship with the patient using a collaborative approach and perhaps utilising guided self-help approaches, incorporating skills derived from cognitive behaviour therapy and its allies, are likely to be more beneficial (and more practical given the time restrictions we have to contend with).

Before getting into specific approaches we need to have an understanding of the therapeutic relationship.

CULTIVATING AN EFFECTIVE RELATIONSHIP – ALL THAT IS REALLY NEEDED?

In Chapter 3 we discussed the importance of listening and the use of 'scissor questioning'. The development of an effective relationship does not usually pose too many problems but knowledge of the topics covered below may be of use should this not be the case.

Accurate empathy – reflective listening

'Stepping oneself into'

We all know of the need to be empathic: to 'step oneself into' the other person's situation. Sometimes the situation can be pretty dire and we need to remember that if empathy is like going into the depths of a person's psychological well, it is very important to hold on very tight to the rope! There is nothing wrong with looking after ourselves in all of this and it is imperative that we do so.

Being empathic is *so, so, so* important if we are to be of any use at all. In subsequent chapters we discuss specific tools to promote change, yet none of them will be helpful unless there is a foundation of empathy to build upon. So how do we show empathy? We read about Carl Rogers' 'unconditional positive regard' in Chapter 1. He described accurate empathy as involving skilful reflective listening that clarifies and amplifies the person's own experiences and meaning, without imposing the counsellor's own material. When we are being empathic we find ourselves mirroring the individual's posture and speak in a similar tone. We employ **reflective listening**; to show that we have heard what has been said we reflect it back. We can do this by repeating, rephrasing or paraphrasing.

Example of reflective listening

> Patient: 'I feel there is nothing to get up for since my family has moved out.'
> Professional: 'You have lost your sense of purpose [pause].'

Notice that there is no question mark at the end of the professional's statement. This means that the intonation of the voice is going down and implies understanding. Most reflective listening statements will be like this (intonation going down and not up). After a further chunk of reflective listening we can use summarising statements.

Example of summarising statement

> 'So all the financial problems and arguments have taken a toll on your relationship; you have become very low indeed and sometimes question whether life is worth living [pause].'

Accurate reflections will only happen if we have listened carefully. When we do this well, the patient feels like we have desired to understand his or her perspective. This allows the building of a working therapeutic alliance.

Quite often, this is all that needs to happen. In general practice, we often see people adjusting to a life crisis, change or loss and while the emotional dust is settling we can provide support and monitoring and at the same time employ reflective listening. If the dust does not settle, then a more structured approach or onward referral might be appropriate.

Reflective listening: a 5-minute review

(From Jeff Allison.[2])

What is it?

A statement designed to convey understanding about what someone has said.

Do I do this already?

Yes, you already do this in normal, everyday conversation – everyone does! Look out for it when watching television or listening to radio, sitting on a train or in a restaurant – it's everywhere. And when you do hear it, listen for the response.

It makes a difference

Consider the difference between these two statements:

> Practitioner A: 'Yes, I understand your concerns.'

> Practitioner B: 'Your main concern about the pain in your knee is that it's made worse by your weight which, in your own words, is "excessive" and that until you find a way to reduce your weight the problem is likely to continue.'

Which of these statements best conveys understanding to the patient?

So how do I do it?

➤ Pay full attention to what you're hearing when the patient is talking. Focus as though your very life depended on you remembering every word.
➤ Try not to think of what to say next while the patient is still speaking.
➤ Imagine you can actually see the words – as in a cartoon speech bubble in a newspaper.
➤ Imagine, also, that you're grabbing the key words or phrases as they emerge and ordering them in your hands – as if you're being dealt a hand of cards. Sort the 'cards'. Ask yourself, 'What's important here? What could I use, now?'
➤ Make a statement, like a mini-summary, of what's been said and your understanding of it (your voice tone goes down at the end, to avoid it sounding like a question).

➤ In your statement use the important 'cards'. You might use some now, and keep others for a later time.
➤ Also consider reflecting the sentiment behind the words, the essence of it. Ask yourself things like, 'What is the patient really getting at?'
➤ Don't rush.
➤ Offer your statement and listen, again, for the response.

Some examples – Table 11.1

The patient's words <u>underlined</u> are the 'cards'. There are some blank reflective responses for you to complete yourself.

TABLE 11.1 Reflective listening

	Patient says	My response	Comment
No. 1	I am having a lot of trouble <u>sleeping</u> in this <u>hospital</u>.	Something's keeping you awake on the ward.	I chose to reflect both cards, as an invitation for her to explain what the difficulty might be.
	It's not so much <u>worrying</u> about things; it's the <u>noise</u>, and the sound of other <u>sick</u> <u>people</u>.	It's true; these hospitals aren't the quietest of places.	I wanted to show that I appreciated what the experience of being a patient was like. I chose not to explore her worries as she indicated that wasn't the most pressing issue.
	Last night this man sounded like he was dying.	?	
No. 2	I <u>don't know</u> whether to have the operation, because I'll be on <u>crutches for 12 months</u>.	It's not like it will be all over when you come out of theatre.	I decided to reflect the concern about being disabled for 12 months.
	That's right, sometimes I think I should just <u>take the risk</u>, and be very <u>careful</u> with my ankle.	You might decide to take a chance.	Reflected the first card and not the second.
	But then if I trip on this ankle, or even just turn on it too much, I'll be completely crippled.	?	

(cont.)

	Patient says	My response	Comment
No. 3	I would like to have this sorted out now, because I am in so much pain that I think I had better stop working.	This pain is getting serious for you.	I decided to focus on one card and it's the most important thing: the pain.
	Yes, it's really serious, and I think I can't carry on like this; I can hardly get out of bed in the morning.	There are times that you feel so disabled that it's difficult to get up.	I focused on how serious it was and the struggle in getting out of bed.
	My wife found me on my knees in tears yesterday and she said I had to come up here and get this sorted out.	?	
No. 4	I don't like the side-effects and this makes me all fat.	The side-effects are bothering you, and you don't want to put on weight.	I decided to add no new material, just to show this patient that I had heard her. I picked out the two most important cards. This encouraged her to continue.
	So I can't win, because if I leave out the drug, I'm taking my chances.	You're caught in the middle, and you're not sure which way to go.	I went further than what she actually said. I captured her dilemma (You're caught in the middle) and emphasised uncertainty about what she might do.
	Well, maybe I can change my diet and keep on the tablets. I don't know.	?	

Therapeutic alliance

(From Patricia Hughes and Ian Kerr. [3])

This is where we establish a rational agreement or contract with our patient, which supports the work we do together. This is often obvious and easy to achieve for simple problems such as 'I've got a sore throat doctor' but if the patient's needs are more 'long term and complex' the therapeutic alliance can become disturbed by wishes and expectations of the patient and/or the doctor. These may or may not be fully conscious. The therapeutic alliance will be affected by the transference and countertransference originally described by Freud and so relevant to our everyday relationships. Very little time and attention is given to these issues in general medical training but an awareness of them is essential if we are to have healthy and productive relationships with our patients. This is especially true where we or our patients have experienced complicated or traumatic previous relationships or unstable attachment formation (*see* Chapter 1– Attachment theory).

Transference[3]

'The unconscious transference of feelings and attitudes from a person or situation in the past onto a person or situation in the present.'

There is a 'projection' of an aspect or wished for/needed aspect of a previously experienced relationship to the other person (health professional in this context). The transference projection is a communication of the individual's needs that cannot be verbally expressed. If the inappropriate feelings dominate the relationship and impede the work to be done then recognising the transference feelings as an unconscious agenda for the patient will help in understanding what the patient wants and expects and can help us in planning clinical management. Dynamic psychotherapy aims to resolve the transference; it promotes bringing reflection and thought to bear on his or her feelings rather than enactment of his or her expectations. However, it is more important for the non-specialist to be aware of transference issues and manage them appropriately. Overtly challenging the patient's feelings is often counterproductive as it can lead to humiliation of the patient and damage the positive aspects of the working relationship. An example would be where there is an inappropriate projection of affection. It would be important to develop strict boundaries so that the patient does not feel that affection is being reciprocated or that the fantasies can have a place in the real world. We need to promote a secure, boundaried and calm environment with the setting of clear limits in treatment. It is important that the patient feels 'held'; that their feelings and problems are being acknowledged and taken seriously and that the working relationship is reasonably stable and predictable. Someone with an immature personality with dependency and emotional instability issues is likely to become emotionally distressed when there is cancellation of a routine, planned appointment with no prior warning. This might increase risk.

Tranference in reverse[3]
We also bring 'emotional baggage' to our present relationships . . .
. . . and there will be some situations that will trigger unthinking reactions at the expense of thoughtful clinical management. It is important to recognise our own preconceptions.

BOX 11.1 CASE STUDY

A woman on my list with a history of childhood trauma, unstable relationships, emotional instability and depressive episodes told me that I was the first doctor she could really talk to, tried to see me more frequently (often unnecessarily) and started asking me to phone her more often after morning surgery. She said it would be beneficial to meet more often. Her behavioural 'nudges' made me aware of a possible transference issue; that a previously needed aspect of a relationship was being projected. At other times she would accuse me of not caring whether she lived or died. Here she was projecting a past scenario where she was neglected and at risk. My recognition of these transferences allowed me to remain calm and supportive while not retaliating to her accusations. At the same time I was able to inform my receptionist colleagues that they must not make promises that I would always call her back (unless there was a specific new medical development). I was able to acknowledge her difficulties while firmly clarifying my availability and agreeing the next appointment time. I ensured there was always a chaperone present for any physical examinations.

If I had refused to see this lady again she would have engaged in 'doctor-hopping' as she had done in years gone by, never establishing a therapeutic alliance. With some solution-focused questioning (see later) I had learned of her impressive artistic talent. Severing our doctor–patient relationship would have put an end to our discussion of these skills (more interesting than warts and chest infections! – selfish I know).

Discussion with colleagues and psychological supervision might just help bring these issues into conscious awareness.

Countertransference[3]

The response of a person to another's unconscious transference communications.

These feelings evoked in us can be a useful guide to the patient's expectations of the relationship. Awareness of a transference-countertransference process can allow for a thoughtful response and plan on our part rather than an unthinking reaction. We can feel confused and despairing when we have painful states of mind projected onto us. It is important to reflect and use the support of our colleagues.

Secure base

In Chapter 5, we considered how those people who take drugs to 'get by' often have emotionally unstable personalities as a result of unstable early attachments. Common personality characteristics were listed. For these people, there was a lack of a 'secure base' in childhood. From the work of Jeremy Holmes,[4] a basic tenet in the management of this patient group is the provision of a secure base. This is about consistency and reliability. As we are dealing with parenting damaged 'children', our approach needs to be consistent and understanding while maintaining firm boundaries as discussed above.

REFERENCES

1. Malan DH. *Individual Psychotherapy and the Science of Psychodynamics.* 2nd ed. Hodder Arnold; 1995.
2. Jeff Allison training. Available at: www.jeffallison.co.uk
3. Hughes P, Kerr I. Transference and countertransference in communication between doctor and patient. *Advances in Psychiatric Treatment.* 2000; 6: 57–64.
4. Holmes J. Psychotherapeutic approaches to the management of severe personality disorder in general psychiatric settings. *CPD Bulletin Psychiatry.* 1999; 1(2): 35–41.

CHAPTER 12

Psychological tools: promoting change in a specific area

In this chapter we learn techniques that promote change in a specific area. These can be used for any behaviour that has an influence on health such as stopping smoking, taking more exercise or engagement in an activity that will help in the moving away from unsatisfactory circumstances (examples given in next chapter). Its application is only limited by our imagination.

> Q: 'How many psychiatrists does it take to change a light bulb?'
> A: 'One . . . but the light bulb has to want to change!!'

You may have noticed that people are not light bulbs. When it comes to change, light bulbs are rather all or nothing – on or off. This is interesting because we often hear health professionals referring to people as if they are light bulbs – 'Oh they don't want to change . . . they'll never change'. However, when humans come to changing something in their lives, there are degrees of wanting to change. There is ambivalence: being in two minds about change.

STAGES OF CHANGE

DiClemente and Prochaska introduced the 'Stages of Change' model.[1] They noted the six stages of change individuals used to change their troubled behaviour: **precontemplation, contemplation, preparation, action, maintenance, and termination** – *see* Figure 12.1. People were found to be using different processes at different times. During the precontemplation phase there was no intention to take action. During the contemplation phase there was an intention to take action. Preparation involved taking some behavioural steps to achieve this. During the action phase the behaviour was changed for less than six months. Maintenance meant that the behaviour had been changed for more than six months. Termination meant that overt behaviour would never return, and there was complete confidence that the person could cope without fear of relapse.

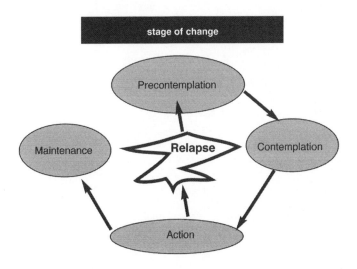

FIGURE 12.1 Stages of change

Since the development of this model there has been a lot of research into how we can help move people through the stages of change.

The material that follows has been adapted from the work of Rollnick and Miller.[2–4]

READY, WILLING AND ABLE – MOTIVATIONAL INTERVIEWING TECHNIQUES

For a change to occur it needs to be given some degree of **importance** by the individual and there needs to be a degree of **confidence** in achieving the change. Figure 12.2 illustrates how the larger the amount of importance and confidence, the more likely it is that change will occur – that the **action** phase will be realised.

To promote change we need the consultation to have the feel of a dance and not of a wrestling match

Imagine an activity holiday based on the shores of the 'River of Change'. Two couples decide to go boating using identical rowing boats. **Confrontational**

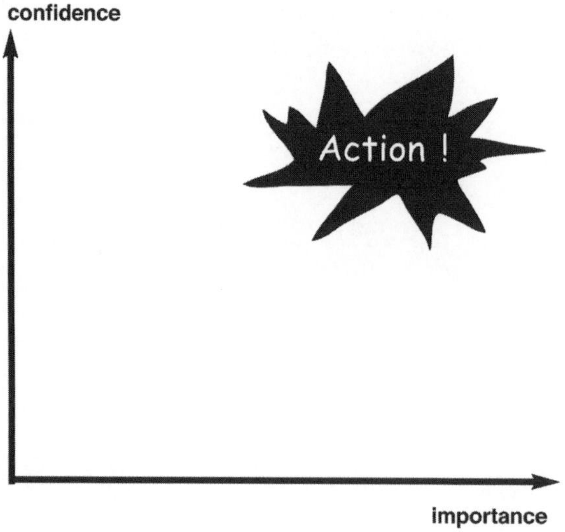

confidence

Action !

importance

FIGURE 12.2 Importance and confidence

CLARE decides that she knows enough about the river not to require oars; that the tidal and weather conditions will go unchanged and that they will adequately propel their boat using hands and feet. This couple quickly find that they are going in the wrong direction and find it hard to cope with the changing tides and wind direction; they are inefficient and disorganised; they become frustrated with each other and end up wrestling on the boat. They really don't enjoy the trip and would have been better off staying at home. The other couple recognise the need for oars and their boat is much more responsive to their actions; they have more power and direction. The couple are thrilled with the distance they travel and the experiences they share. In fact they end up dancing together. The rest of this chapter builds on the fact that being a **Confrontational CLARE** leads to wrestling and going nowhere whereas using our **OARS** brings us to dancing and the achievement of great things.

Wrestling – building resistance to change; being a Confrontational CLARE
Certain interviewing characteristics will get in the way of exploring ambivalence. Patients value advice but they do not like being preached to. Confrontation leads to the patient who feels two ways about something arguing for the opposite. If we increase the confrontation, there will be an increase in 'yes . . . but' statements from the patient. As a person argues on behalf of one position, he or she becomes more committed to it (self-perception theory) – they 'talk themselves into . . . '. So being confrontational will increase **resistance** to change. The letters in confrontational **CLARE**'s name can act as a useful aide

memoire to the other resistance building interviewing features: the things that make a consultation more of a wrestle than a dance.

CLARE

➤ Criticising, shaming, blaming.
➤ Labelling – what the person 'is' or 'has'.
➤ Arguing for change.
➤ Being perceived as being in a hurry/Rush.
➤ Assuming the Expert role as if we have all the answers and 'I know what is best for you'.

Dancing – using OARS

OARS

O – Open Questions.
A – Affirming.
R – Reflective Listening.
S – Summarising.

In looking at the importance for change we need to develop discrepancy – the mismatch between current behaviour and values for the future. In Chapter 2 we read about Cognitive Dissonance Theory and here we are trying to develop/enhance the dissonance pressure (discomfort brought about by the mismatch between values and current behaviour). By developing and elaborating discrepancy we enhance the perceived importance of change. We need to work in a way that promotes the patient voicing arguments for change; this involves using **OARS** – *see* Figure 12.3.

The parts of the **OARS** that need to be in the water most of the time to allow smooth passage down the river of change are the use of open questions

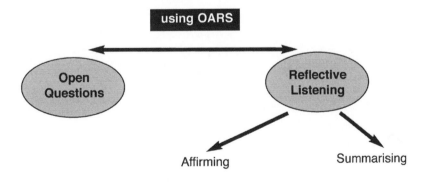

FIGURE 12.3 Using OARS

(as discussed in Chapter 3) and reflective listening. These allow us to focus on the concerns and perspective of the individual. If you haven't yet read the five-minute reflective listening review in the previous chapter, please invest some time on it now before moving forward with this chapter.

WILLING – IMPORTANCE FOR CHANGE, EXPLORING AMBIVALENCE

The amount we want to change will wax and wane – so perhaps we're more like light bulbs with dimmer switches! Rollnick and Miller[2-4] have developed Motivational Interviewing as a method for enhancing intrinsic motivation to change. This is a great tool that gets us away from preaching and confrontation and instead leads the patient to tell us why they feel they should change. Although it has been traditionally considered for use in the field of substance misuse, we can apply it to any change situation. We will be using their work and blending it slightly with other solution-focused approaches.

Ambivalence is normal and means the holding of conflicting thoughts about something – feeling two ways about something (e.g. cigarettes, heroin use, a neighbour). Ambivalence has implications for how to interview someone to bring them closer to change. It seems pointless knowing that smoking, being overweight and eating cat food is unhealthy behaviour unless we know how to communicate in a way that promotes healthy change.

Getting onto the dance floor

But how do we get onto the dance floor?

1 Easy – when the person really wants to dance and asks you:

> Patient: Doctor, I've come today to talk about my weight/drinking/smoking.

2 Not so easy – When the music is perfect for you but you are not sure what the other person feels about it. There are two potential situations.

   a **Feedback of results or review of a chronic disease/condition**
     This might be the case when we need to feedback clinical information that is related to lifestyle factors, e.g. blood results and alcohol, body mass index and weight issues. Alternatively, we might be holding a chronic disease review, e.g. diabetes/asthma, and wish to review the factors that influence control over the condition, e.g. use of inhalers, diet, smoking.

> Practitioner: [. . .] is sometimes linked with, or caused by [. . .] I wonder if we could talk briefly about whether that might apply to you?
> Practitioner: How do you feel about the amount you drink?

Practitioner: Have you ever considered whether getting more exercise might improve control of your diabetes?

Practitioner: What would you like to talk about? Changing your diet, getting more exercise, or is there something else that seems more important for you today?

b **Opportunistic**

We need to employ '**constructive listening**' to gauge the person's readiness for the dance.

During constructive listening we are listening for '**cues**'. Let us take the common example of someone coming to see their GP with a chesty cough and feeling grotty. The doctor is listening to her chest when the conversation goes like this:

Mrs Fume: 'Well, I am still smoking doctor.'

This is a cue and tells us that there may be a degree of contemplation going on in the head of Mrs Fume – some consideration of a possible link between smoking and her chest problem. The doctor can take her lead. He might wish to put this cue on the back burner and deal with the immediate problem of the possible chest infection and discuss the management of this before returning to the cue and bringing it to the front burner – or he might like to use the cue straight away.

If Mrs Fume had not mentioned her smoking it would have been routine for the doctor to have enquired about her smoking status – this would have been a closed question ('Do you smoke, Mrs Fume?').

Once she had answered with a 'yes' the doctor has the opportunity to start dancing. Asking permission to discuss a lifestyle issue will help in reducing resistance.

Doctor: 'Would it be OK to explore the topic of smoking a little? . . .' [if answers yes/OK . . .]

'Perhaps you could help me to see the big picture Mrs Fume . . . how do you feel about the smoking?' . . . [*reflective listening, reflective listening, reflective listening + + +*] . . .

'What do you enjoy about smoking?' . . . [*reflective listening, reflective listening, reflective listening + + + +*] . . .

'I wonder if there is another side of the coin for you . . . what is the not so good side?' . . . [*reflective listening, reflective listening, reflective listening*]

So during this smooth dance we are exploring ambivalence, looking at the pros and cons of her behaviour, the two ways she feels about it. As well as being person centred, the approach is also directive in that we can selectively reflect back information, giving extra weight to **change talk** – speech that is directed towards the desired kind of change. We can also encourage elaboration of any change talk.

There are some other helpful ways of collecting information and exploring ambivalence. We can use a decisional balance table and scaling questions relating to the importance of change.

Importance scale

> Doctor: 'On a scale of one to 10 where 10 means that it is the most important thing in your life to stop smoking and one means that it is not at all important to you to give up any cigarettes ever . . . where would you be now?'

Tip for scales

Always make one out of 10 very extreme – in this example the patient is unlikely to score herself at one when this would signify 'not at all important to you to give up any cigarettes ever'. The fact that she has mentioned smoking to you indicates that she has contemplated a link between smoking and her health. In the case of a chronically depressed person seeing you at the surgery I might indicate 'so low that cannot even manage to get out of bed' – as they are here in the surgery they will not score themselves at one.

Plotting herself on the scale, either mentally or with paper and pen (however low she scores her importance), provides an opportunity – *see* Figure 12.4.

> Doctor: 'That's interesting . . . so there is a big enough part of you to score you at three – can you tell me about this part of you?' – [reflective listening, elaboration]
> 'Why are you at three and not zero?'– [*reflective listening, elaboration*]
> 'What would it take for you to go from three to four?' – [*reflective listening, elaboration*]

Who knows what she will tell us next. Her reasons might be different from the next person. People change things for their own reasons in their own time. They may or may not be health reasons; she might like to protect her cat from the effects of passive smoking! We need to encourage her to **elaborate** on anything she says, so that the 3/10 score ends up feeling more substantial – a bigger 3/10:

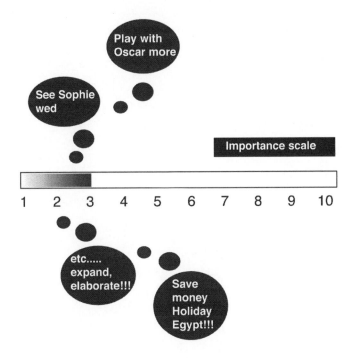

FIGURE 12.4 Importance scale

Mrs Fume: 'Well it's bad for your health doctor.' [write it on the scale]

Doctor: 'You are worried that it could make you ill.'

Mrs Fume: 'Yes, I don't want to get lung cancer doctor.'

Doctor: 'It's important to you to avoid lung cancer . . . [*pause – a chance for her to elaborate*] . . . how would you prefer things to be in the future in a life without lung cancer' [*turn everything into a positive alternative*].

Mrs Fume: 'To have healthy lungs I suppose.'

Doctor: 'Yes, and I guess you might know this already but the good news is that your risk of lung cancer drops considerably after just a few years of no smoking [*so, following her lead, we can introduce some positive health advice*] . . . How would you know if your lungs were more healthy – what would you notice?'

Mrs Fume: 'I wouldn't get so short of breath.'

Doctor: 'So you would breathe more easily' [*turning to the positive again – it is positive suggestions that 'stick'*].

Tip

Turn everything into a positive – positive suggestions stick.

> Mrs Fume: 'Yes.'
> Doctor: 'What impact would that have on your life?'
> Mrs Fume: 'I would be able to keep up with the grandchildren for longer.'
> Doctor: '... What are they called? ... When do you see them? ... What would you want to be doing with them?' ... etc ... [*elaborate, elaborate, elaborate!*]
> Doctor: 'What else?' [*what else is a great question when we are trying to elaborate*]; 'Why else have you got that element of importance?'
> Mrs Fume: 'Would save some money?'
> Doctor: 'How much do you spend?' ... 'So you would save £x' ... 'What would you spend it on instead?' ... 'Where would you go on holiday?' ... etc [*expand, expand, expand!*]

What is great is that we are finding out some interesting things about our patient – the things they like to do etc. They feel like we are interested in them. We feel like we have something to talk to them about the next time they present with a 'boring' problem.

Summarise

Then we need to summarise why Mrs Fume wants to stop smoking (to the degree that she wants to stop).

> Doctor: 'Thank you for taking the time to discuss your smoking with me. I can see that you enjoy the company of your work colleagues when you go outside for a smoke and that when you first inhale you feel calm as your craving subsides ... and it also looks like you want to have healthy lungs so that you can run more with Sophie and Oscar on the beach ... instead of developing lung cancer you want to live to see Sophie get married ... and you have always wanted to see the pyramids and after being off the cigarettes for two years you will be able to afford to take Fred there on a second honeymoon.'

You can see that we have acknowledged the benefits she sees smoking has for her but we have selectively summarised the elaborated material relating to change. All of this information came from her and is therefore likely to be accepted by her.

Affirmations

Particularly when resistance is high, it can be helpful to offer some positive affirmations along the way.

> 'I can see that you have a real sense of responsibility towards your grandchildren and that they really enjoy your involvement.'

When a person has come for the first time to discuss their difficult and sensitive problem:

> 'It must have been a big step coming here today.'

ABLE – CONFIDENCE – SELF-EFFICACY

It is often the case that when importance is big enough the individual will find an avenue for change that they believe they can successfully travel down. Here we aim to develop such self-efficacy/confidence. Interestingly, if an avenue for change is not found then Anna Freud's defence mechanisms (*see* Chapter 1) come into play.

➤ Denial – 'It's not really that bad'.
➤ Rationalisation – 'I did not want it anyway'.
➤ Projection – 'It's not my problem, it's theirs'.

Open questions

> 'How might you go about making this change?'
> 'What would be a good first step?'
> 'What obstacles do you foresee, and how might you deal with them?'

Confidence scale

> Doctor: 'So, thanks for that . . . I feel like I understand the bigger picture now . . . But can you imagine for me before you go . . . a scale of confidence? On this one to 10 scale, one signifies that there is no way you could give up any cigarettes ever [*very extreme, remember*] . . . and 10 indicates that it would be really easy to give up all your fags tomorrow . . . where would you be now?'
> Mrs Fume: 'Um . . . four I reckon.'
> Doctor: 'Tell me about this chunk of confidence . . . how come you score four and not three?'
> Mrs Fume: 'Well, I've done it before.'
> Doctor: 'You've done it before' . . . 'How did you manage to stop last time?' . . . elaborate, elaborate!! [*remember different things work for different people*]

'What else, what else, what else?'

Mrs Fume: 'I've managed to cope with other difficult changes in my life.'

Doctor: 'The strengths you used in the past could help with overcoming this hurdle. . . . What did it take to cope with past difficulties?' [*Establishing her resources*]

Mrs Fume: 'Willpower I suppose, also I've got some good friends.' [*so she has internal resources, e.g. willpower, and she has external resources, e.g. friends*].

Tip

Resources can be internal or external. Get a history of resources.

Doctor: 'Willpower . . . that's interesting . . . how long have you recognised that you have willpower?'

[*Get a history of her resources. When they became noticeable to her, what they have helped with in her life – makes a change from focusing on problems and vulnerabilities, doesn't it?*]

'What else, what else etc.'

Summarise

Summarise again.

'Who would be least surprised?'

This is a wonderful question. Not 'who would be most surprised if you stopped smoking' but . . .

Doctor: 'Mrs Fume . . . you have been on this earth for 56 years and I guess you have known many people. Can you tell me which person . . . might be someone from your past . . . or someone currently in your life . . . can you tell me which person would be least surprised if you stopped smoking?'

Mrs Fume: 'Ooooohh . . . that's a difficult one . . . I don't know.'

Doctor: 'Well if you did know . . . what would you tell me?' [*cheeky! But do not give up . . . get a name!*]

Mrs Fume: 'Mrs Pencil . . . my art teacher when I was at secondary school.'

Doctor: 'Ok . . . so what did she know about you. What did she know that would make her least surprised if you gave up smoking?'

Mrs Fume: 'She knew I was determined; I confided in her about troubles at home and despite this I got a grade A.' [*more strengths and resources*]

Doctor: 'Well, thanks for that.' [*summarise again – emphasis on change talk*].

READY

Change might be very important and there might be the confidence to bring it about but is it given high enough priority at this time?

How do we know if they are ready for change and that the time is right for strengthening their commitment? There will be more change talk (speech that is directed towards the desired kind of change) and less resistance. Readiness for change is not likely to be a sudden happening; there may be preparation for change – new growth, even though there are a few dead leaves of ambivalence left in the garden to be swept away. Despite a lot of change talk there may be a lot of dead leaves about – tread carefully or you will damage the new shoots that lie beneath them! If we assume readiness too soon we might damage this new growth.

At this point we need to get the balance right; we don't want to be too directive yet we need to encourage some direction.

Summarise

Start by summarising what we have learnt so far. Include all the reasons for change that have been covered along with acknowledgement of ambivalence. Then:

'How do you really feel about [ ]. How ready for change are you?'

Readiness scale

'If one was "not ready" and 10 was "ready" what score would you give yourself?'
'You gave yourself a score of six. Why six and not five?'
'What would need to happen for you to move up to seven?'

Setting goals

'What is the next step?'
'Where do we go from here?'
'What changes, if any, are you thinking of making?'
'How would you like things to be different?'
'What is it that you want to change?'
'What do you think would be the first step?'

There may need to be some priority setting if there is more than one goal.

Checking the goal is realistic

'How might your life be different if you reached the goal?'
'What might go wrong with the plan?'

Giving information

Ask permission first:

'I have some ideas about this which may or may not be relevant; do you want to hear them?'

If you are asked for advice:

'Well, we are all different and what works for one person will not work for everyone. I would not want to tell you what to do as you are the expert on you and I would not want to interfere with any of the ideas you may already have. Maybe you would like to hear of some of the options that have been helpful to other people and you could see which, if any, might be helpful to you.'

Brainstorming

Doctor: 'So let's think about what it might take to stop smoking again; let's think of any way at all that it might happen, as many different ways as possible.'
[*Elaborate and explore the different possible ways*]

Brainstorm possible strategies and consider the pros and cons for those strategies; draw on the individual's internal and external resources.

Agree a plan

Summarise the plan.

'Is this what you want to do?'

Hopefully the answer will be yes. A different answer will require discussion of what was incorrect within the plan summary. Further reflective listening and exploration of ambivalence may need to take place.

This might seem a lot of work. However, you can see that it can be chunked down into smaller parts and does not all have to be done at once.

Research into these techniques tells us that it works. Scaling questions help to break extreme, polarised, black and white (light-bulb) thinking. We learn that there is more to our patients than their problems. We will use scaling questions again later.

REFERENCES

1. Prochaska JO, DiClemente CC. Stages and processes of self-change of smoking: toward an integrative model of change. *J Consult Clin Psychol.* 1983; **51**: 390–5.
2. Miller WR, Rollnick S. *Motivational Interviewing: Preparing People for Change.* 2nd ed. New York: Guilford Press; 2002.
3. Rollnick S, Mason P, Butler C. *Health Behavior Change: A Guide for Practitioners.* Churchill Livingstone; 1999.
4. Rollnick S, Dunn C. *Rapid Reference to Lifestyle and Behavior Change (Rapid Reference).* Mosby; 2003.

FURTHER TRAINING

www.stephenrollnick.com
www.jeffallison.co.uk

CHAPTER 13

Psychological tools: tools for general use

In Part Two, where appropriate, we considered psychological approaches for specific problem areas. In this chapter we focus on approaches that:
➤ provide us with some emotional protection in the face of relentless presenting problems
➤ have multiple applications for problems along the psychological-physical spectrum
➤ are easily chunked for short encounters

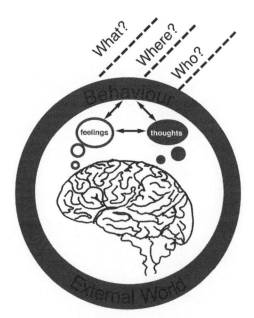

FIGURE 13.1 Thoughts, feelings, behaviours

➤ link to signposting to other resources (to help with our growing capacity issue).

To achieve this, we will explore a framework developed from solution-focused and motivational interviewing techniques overlapping with cognitive behaviour therapy, problem-solving approaches as well as systemic and family therapies. Providers of further training are listed at the end of the chapter. There are a number of refreshing elements to all of this that help protect us in our work and aid our enjoyment of it.

You will start working with the person rather than the problem; look for resources rather than deficits and treat the individual as the expert in all aspects of their life. This sounds quite different from the usual medical encounters we have – and it is. Steve de Shazer and his wife Insoo Kim Berg were the primary developers of the Solution-Focused Brief Therapy approach which, though simple to learn, can be a challenge to practise if we let our traditional problem-orientated learning get in the way.

You will notice a shift in responsibilities and this will bring with it a sense of relief. This will happen by adopting the view that the individual in front of you is actually the expert when it comes to them and that they have the resources to bring about change. There is an emphasis on the patient resolving his or her problems. Patients specify their own goals for treatment and the practitioner assists with this. This approach may not initially be welcomed by patients who want their problems to be solved for them. However, the approach avoids getting caught up in a discussion that there is nothing that can be done and is a great way for the practitioner to set their stall out and lay down appropriate boundaries, particularly for heart-sink situations; when the problems are long-standing and complex.

The approach is easy to learn but can be difficult to perform as you will be required to get into a new mind-set and be willing to give it a go. The more practice, the easier it gets.

EXPLORING THOUGHTS, FEELING AND BEHAVIOURS

Thoughts, feelings and behaviours influence each other. A change in one part of a system will influence other parts of the system. We need to give this some consideration before moving on.

The way we think affects the way we feel and the way we think and feel affects the way we behave – *see* Figure 13.1.

Feelings (or moods) are best described using one word.

Examples of feelings/moods:

Depressed; Anxious; Angry; Guilty; Ashamed; Sad;
Embarrassed; Excited; Frightened; Irritated; Insecure
Proud; Mad; Panicky; Frustrated; Nervous; Disgusted
Hurt; Cheerful; Disappointed; Enraged; Scared; Happy
Loving; Humiliated

Our thoughts (cognitions) come as sentences or images. Mental health problems are often associated with extreme negative thoughts. Types of thinking 'errors' were discussed in Chapter 2. Feelings of anxiety are usually associated with thoughts concerning the possibility of future misfortune – 'what if' thoughts.

Examples of thoughts and their impact on mood and behaviours include the following.

1 **Thought**: What if I fall over when I do my talk?
   Mood: Anxious
   Behaviour: Avoid doing talks
2 **Thought**: She is rude . . . she is insulting me.
   Mood: Irritated
   Behaviour: Physical violence
3 **Thought**: She does not find me interesting . . . I bore everybody.
   Mood: Sad
   Behaviour: Drinking bottle of whisky
4 **Thought**: She seems shy . . . she is probably too uncomfortable to look at me.
   Mood: Caring
   Behaviour: Initiate conversation

We learnt in Chapter 2 that our mood states and thinking content will have bearing on our behaviours and activity choices. Our thinking styles are rooted in our core beliefs (*see* Chapter 1), which are formed as a result of early relationships and events.

Cognitive behaviour therapy aims to help people identify their extreme negative thinking patterns and to get a more balanced view (thought) about situations. It often involves diarising the thoughts and feelings that are associated with different situations and then looking at evidence for and against any extreme thinking. There is good evidence that self-help CBT is effective. The following are examples of researched, accessible packages:

➤ The MoodGym programme available free at www.moodgym.anu.edu.au
➤ The CBT self-help manual – *Mind Over Mood* by Dennis Greenberger, Christine Padesky (Guilford Publications, 1995).

Formal CBT is likely to be too time-consuming for the primary care health practitioner. However, it is useful to educate the patient about the relationship between thoughts, feelings and behaviours.

When we consider behaviour it is useful to think of our relationship to the environment/social system in terms of:

➤ what we do
➤ where we do it
➤ who we do it with.

Just as certain styles of thinking will impact on our mood, doing certain things with certain people in certain places will impact on our thoughts and feelings. Interpersonal Therapy (IPT) has been studied in the treatment of bulimia nervosa. This is an approach that focuses on relationships and their effect on our mental health. In IPT treatment of bulimia, talk about food is not permitted, yet research has confirmed that IPT has therapeutic long-term results equivalent to CBT.[1–3] It is also the case that IPT is as effective as CBT in the treatment of depression. These findings highlight the strength of influence our relationships have over our mental health. Many mental health problems are rooted in low self-esteem which is affected by the quality of our relationships.

The 'BATHE' technique

In their very practical book, *The Fifteen Minute Hour: Therapeutic Talk In Primary Care*,[4] Stuart and Lieberman help primary care practitioners apply CBT principles in their brief patient encounters. They introduce the 'BATHE' technique. They advocate using the technique in all consultations. 'BATHE' stands for Background, Affect, Trouble, Handling, Empathy:

B – Background

> 'What is going on in your life?'
> 'Tell me what's been happening since I saw you last?'
> 'What was going on in your life about that time?'

If the patient responds with 'nothing', Stuart and Lieberman advise us to persist with the technique, perhaps by repeating the word 'nothing?' to encourage further thought by the patient. If they continue with the premise that nothing has been happening, then it is appropriate to continue with the next item of the technique and enquire how it makes the patient feel not having anything going on in their life. Not making further enquiry risks reinforcing somatisation (*see* Chapter 8) as the patient is not given the opportunity to form links between emotional and physical symptomatology.

A – Affect (feelings)

> 'How do you feel about that?'
> 'How does that make you feel?'

T – Trouble (cognitive – thought assessment)

> 'What about the situation troubles you the most?'

H – Handling (behavioural assessment)

> 'How are you handling that?'
> 'How could you handle that?'

Implied in the question is the suggestion that the patient is capable of managing the situation.

E – Empathy

> 'That must be very difficult for you.'

Legitimises the patient's reaction.
    Reflective listening as outlined in Chapter 11 is used.

Four options

Stuart and Lieberman also provide four options for dealing with a troubling situation. It can be helpful to discuss these with our patients:

Leaving it

Encourage the patient to consider the likelihood of best and worst possible outcomes along with strategies to help deal with any consequences.

Changing it

Define what needs to be different – see below; consider the resources and strategies that are required to bring about change.

Accepting it as it is

Considering 'exceptions' can help with this – aspects of the situation that are acceptable/going well. This idea is further developed below.

Identify and develop resources, sources of support and enjoyment to provide an emotional buffer.

Reframing it

Interpreting the situation differently as it is the meaning that we attribute to a situation that determines how we feel about it.

A 'POSITIVE PSYCHOLOGY' FRAMEWORK

Positive psychology is the study of human strengths and virtues. Talking about problems all the time runs the risk of reinforcing the negative emotional state of the patient. The framework we will be exploring during this section of the chapter is summarised in Figure 13.2:

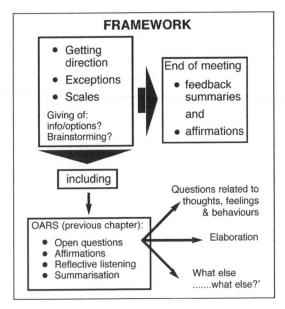

FIGURE 13.2 Psychological tools framework

At first glance this might look rather complicated. However, as we work through the chapter all will become clear. We can chunk it down for use during separate brief encounters as and when we find the appropriate time. I have found 'frequent attending' patients with multiple long-standing complex problems become easier to manage. I have, on some occasions, given some patients an initial longer consultation to get matters under way and to develop some useful momentum. This investment of time (usually an extended meeting at the end of a surgery) then 'sets the scene' for the future, more time-limited encounters to come.

GETTING DIRECTION – A PREFERRED FUTURE

If we were treating raised blood pressure or targeting diabetic blood glucose control, we would have a management goal. This should be no different. We need to explore what the person hopes to achieve, making this as crystal clear as possible. Certain questions help to establish this.

> 'What needs to be different?'
> 'How would we know if things had improved for you?'
> 'If in six months' time life was going well, how would you know?'
> 'What would you see/hear/feel that tells you that you have achieved that?'
> 'How would we know if our time together looking at your issues had been helpful?'

Have you ever noticed that when you buy something, for example, a different car, that you start to notice the same model whenever you are out and about. Opinion has it that this is due to a setting of the brain's 'reticular activating system'. This complex collection of brainstem neurones serves as a point of convergence for signals from the external world and from the interior environment. In other words, it is the part of your brain where the world outside you, and your thoughts and feelings from 'inside' you, meet. The reticular activating system in the brain acts as a filter for information coming in and it does this in a way that is consistent with our beliefs and our goals. By using the above questions and encouraging the individual to elaborate we could be setting the reticular activating system. The person will then begin to notice anything that might be associated with their preferred future. Having a 'purpose' is important. It is more important than being rigid about the 'process' or method of getting there. Being too loyal to a particular plan may leave us 'blinkered', with tunnel vision and we may not notice opportunities that come our way that might guide us towards our goal.

It is useful to expand any information offered. Sometimes the individual has been so engrossed by all their problems that they have not stopped to think about their preferred future (and have forgotten that there is more to them than their problems!). Taking time out to do this can have quite remarkable results.

BOX 13.1 CASE STUDY

A woman joined my patient list. Physical and emotional problems had been overwhelming her family for years. I was feeling extremely pressured by my workload on a particular day when I was asked to phone her. She told me that I needed to help her because everything in her life was awful and that something needed to be done. Having established that there were no immediate risks to anyone I asked her 'what needs to be different?' She did not know what to say for a while. It took a while before she was able to tell me that she did not want to feel so depressed all the time. I was interested to know how she wished to feel instead. She told me she wanted to feel more calm and cheerful more often. Knowing that there were problems of arthritis and marital disharmony I asked her to spend time writing down everything that she wished to be different. I advised her to 'turn everything around' and to elaborate so that we would learn, for example, how being more pain-free would impact on her; what she would be able to do differently without so much pain; how this would make her feel; who would notice her feeling this way; what she would be thinking about instead of the pain. In other words, she was to build up a mental picture of what life would be like. I told her to make an appointment to see me once she had carried out this exercise as it would help us both know where she needed to be going.

She did attend at a later date and told me she had started to feel brighter in herself. She had recognised that, for her, being happier would be associated with spending more time with people who shared the same interests. She had reminded herself of her long-lost interests and had enrolled in an adult education class with a friend. Time away from the home with someone she liked and trusted and achieving at things that she wanted to do for herself were bolstering her self-esteem and mood. Interestingly the distraction was also helping her to manage her arthritis pain. So often, making a change in one area will have positive knock-on effects in other areas.

Great that this lady had started to make inroads into her problems 'just like that' but even if she had just attended with her written notes, we would have developed important direction.

Helping to elaborate and 'turn things' around is crucial. Not feeling so anxious might become feeling more calm. This might allow someone to paint better or phone their gran. Not cutting skin so frequently might become stroking the pet hamster more often. Stroking the hamster might bring about all sorts of helpful thoughts and feelings – and the cat might notice a smile and who knows what will happen next! And what is great is that you did not know that she had pets and now you have some problem-free material to talk about next time. Once the conversation develops, the affect (immediate mood) of the individual often lifts as they begin to talk about the positives.

Table 13.1 offers some questioning tips:

TABLE 13.1 Questioning tips

Thoughts (cognitions)	Feelings (moods)	Behaviours
How will you be thinking if you did that?	If you were thinking about that . . . how would that make you feel?	What would you be doing differently?
In what way would that impact on how you'd be thinking?	If you were doing more [ ] . . . how would that make you feel?	What might that make you do?
What might you be thinking if you were feeling/doing more [ ]?		How will thinking/feeling like that show itself?
		If you were thinking/ feeling like that, who would notice? . . . What would they notice? . . . What would happen then?

If you feel stuck then just remember how thoughts, feelings and behaviours are connected and ask about each accordingly and ask what would happen next. Remember, you can always ask:

What else . . . What else . . . What else . . . What else . . . What else?!!
This can be tricky for patients who have been stuck with their negative cogs (cognitions) going around. Imagining a life without the problem can be different and requires persistence on both the part of the practitioner and the patient. Lots of grease has to be applied to those rusty old alternative 'cogs' that have got stuck down over difficult times. However, the effort is worth it – they will start to turn and a momentum will become established. So when a patient says, 'I don't know what I would be doing', **do not give up**. You could ask:

'Well, if you did know what would you say?' (!)

Consider the wider picture and significant others:

'It is difficult, isn't it? . . . But you did say that Philip would notice you smiling more and would probably give you more hugs. It sounds like he knows you well. If he was sitting here now, what do you think he'd say you would be doing differently?'

Exploring a preferred future can be taken further by asking the '**Miracle Question**':

> 'Imagine you go to bed tonight and while you are asleep a miracle happens . . . I'm not saying I believe in miracles . . . but pretend a miracle happens . . . and this miracle resolves the problem you have. Because you are asleep you won't know the miracle has happened. When you wake up tomorrow how will you find out? What will you notice first of all? . . .'

This then allows exploration of the 'miracle day' from beginning to end with a lot of grease application to very rusty cogs as the thoughts, feelings and behaviours (what, where, who with) are discovered. In Solution-Focused Brief Therapy this can take a whole 50-minute session. We haven't got this time available to us but whether we just get to morning coffee time in the miracle day or expand and elaborate 'what needs to be different', it will have been worth it. We can always leave the patient to give these issues more consideration between consultations.

EXCEPTIONS

Life isn't black and white; there are degrees to everything. Exceptions are when things do not happen, happen less intensely or happen less frequently. Examples of exception questioning:

When are the times that it doesn't happen?
When are the times that it doesn't last as long?
When are the times that it seems to be less intense?
When are the times that you feel better?
When are the times that it bothers you least?
When do you resist the urge to . . .?

We have discussed the importance of empathy. If someone is feeling very desperate, it would not be appropriate to ask, 'Hey, when is life rosy and tickety-boo?'! It would be more appropriate to ask:

> 'Life is obviously very difficult for you at the moment . . . I wondered if you can think of any times over the last few months when although things have been difficult . . . they have been a little less difficult?'

When the patient feels their problems have been acknowledged and that they have been listened to they are more likely to come up with an answer.

BOX 13.2 CASE STUDY

A 15-year-old girl, Anna, had the symptoms and signs of anorexia nervosa. Her body mass index was dangerously low. Her family were worried to the extreme. They were aware of the risk of mortality that came with her condition. The screaming and shouting at the dinner table were having no effect on her eating. This really was a situation where the EE (Expressed Emotion – *see* Chapter 1) level was high within the home and understandably so. How difficult it must be for terrified parents to avoid becoming too over-involved, critical and seemingly hostile when their child is starving herself. I saw Anna alone and asked her what needed to be different. I purposefully kept away from the matter of food and eating. I already knew her weight and biochemical results and the impact her not eating was having. She had seemed in a state of denial (a defence mechanism – *see* Chapter 1). She would not admit to there being a health-threatening eating problem when challenged by her parents. It was time for some problem-free talk. She told me that she wanted some more energy and her reason was so that she could dance again. We spent some time discussing her dance interest, her associated friends. I then asked her whether there had been any periods of time over the preceding two months when she had been able to dance to some degree (an 'exception'). She said there had been two occasions and she described these to me. I asked her to elaborate on what had been different in great detail. As we were running out of time I was able to provide constructive feedback. Feedback provides an opportunity to confirm what has been learnt and also to give a compliment.

'So it sounds like you thoroughly enjoy dance. It has been interesting to hear how you have really achieved at this over the last few years and that it has taken a lot of hard work and commitment, particularly as you have lacked energy. As you say, it has taken willpower and I can see that your willpower has been important to you over the last few years. It has been good to learn that you have some really supportive friends and that being in Lucy's home is where you feel calm; with Lucy in whom you can trust and confide, talk about the things you have done together and think about your future plans together; eating a little of what you like such as bananas, a bit of toast now and then over a few days seemed to help you feel brighter and more energised and able to practise dance a little with Lucy. It is interesting that certain things work for you in your attempt to feel more energised.'

Constructive feedback

When giving constructive feedback:

➤ acknowledge the difficulty of the patient's position

➤ feed back resources

➤ feed back what is working for the patient.

During our chat Anna changed from looking very withdrawn and 'flat' to being more animated. When giving feedback/compliments do not make assumptions; draw from the information presented by the patient – positive suggestions will stick if they make sense to the patient.

A history of resources

Although not outlined in detail above I had obtained a history of Anna's willpower resource:

> 'So you got a dance medal while feeling so drained of energy. What did that take?'
> 'So you have willpower. When was the first time you realised that?'
> 'I know it can be hard to remember these things but what do you reckon?'
> 'Around age 10. Has it been useful to you? How has it helped . . .?'

Some might be tempted to say 'so when you eat, you have more energy – so go and eat more then'. The above approach may have sown enough seeds to allow some 'change-shoots' to start sprouting without the need for any confrontation. People do things for their own reasons and when the time is right for them and not because we tell them to. We will look at this in a little while. If she started to eat a little more, often she would be able to dance more – an offshoot would be that she would not die of starvation though this is not the priority for her right now.

An appropriate way to end the session might be:

> 'Between now and when we next meet perhaps you could notice any other times when you feel a little more energetic. Thanks for coming and I look forward to seeing you next time.'

BOX 13.3 CASE STUDY

A girl with insulin dependent diabetes is erratic with the use of her insulin and her family are despairing. What she wants to be different is for people to be happier at home. There have been times when things have been a bit better. It tends to happen when she has been at her gran's house for a chat. She leaves there feeling better about herself and worthy of good health and fulfilment of her long-term dreams/goals and then takes her insulin. Her family then 'give her a break'. In fact they talk about other things – about going on holiday to France again; this makes her feel happier and more wanted. Her dad notices because she smiles and he then gives her a cuddle – she might then find herself taking her insulin in a more organised way for a few days after that.

BOX 13.4 CASE STUDY

A 54-year-old man has a history of long-standing neck pain and return visits to his doctor for sickness certificates. The doctor has never been convinced that a physical problem existed, particularly as physical tests had been normal. Whatever the cause of the pain, the aim of the professional should be to help the patient lose their symptoms without losing face. Months ago, before the accident that led to his pain, the man worked with a team of people. The doctor felt unsure how to proceed. The following proved useful:

> 'Clearly you have been experiencing a lot of pain. Can you tell me about the times over the last three weeks when the pain, although a problem, has not been quite so bothersome or noticeable?'

The man eventually described being with his young grandchildren on the common kicking a football around. His mind had been distracted; he was thinking of other things and feeling happier. We learnt that distraction by being with people was helpful in managing the pain (and, yes, perhaps being back at work might be the best way of managing the pain and this could be explored at the appropriate time).

End of session

Always give a feedback summary with affirmations (as above – 15-year-old Anna).

You might like to leave things as they are with a plan to meet again. Sometimes this style of communication will have provided enough ingredients for some between-session changes to be cooked up.

Alternatively, you might like to leave a noticing-suggestion after summarisation with affirmation:

'I have an idea of what might be helpful between now and when we next meet – would you like to hear it? I wonder if you might like to notice those times when you have a little more energy so that we can learn more about what is working for you. We could discuss anything you notice next time. How does that sound?'

Document what you have discovered (what needs to be different, strengths and resources) and any agreed task.

SCALING QUESTIONS

These provide an opportunity for breaking the extreme polarised ('black or white') thinking that often occurs in emotional problems. They are also a means for charting progress.

Take someone with chronic low mood.

Q: 'On a scale of 1–10 with 10 representing feeling happy about everything all the time and one representing feeling so low that you cannot even get out of bed, where would you say you are?'

A: 'three'

Q: 'Where on the scale would represent "good enough" do you think . . . or "OK"?'

(*Implied in this question is the fact that it is not normal to be at 10 – to feel happy all the time*)

A: 'seven'

Tip for scales

Remember to make one out of 10 very extreme – lower than you suspect the patient is (easy in this example; the fact that she is here in your room means that she cannot score herself at one because she is obviously not in bed!).

Your questioning will be influenced by the state of the patient – remember empathy is all important. So for a struggling patient one might ask:

'What seems to be stopping things getting worse despite the difficulties you face?'

Or:

'How are you managing to hold things where they are despite such difficulties?'

Or:

'Clearly things have been very difficult; how have you been managing to get out of bed? . . . What has been making you get out of bed? . . . What did that take?'

However, if the patient is a little more buoyant one might ask:

'What is it that has helped you get from one to where you are now?'

Or:

'What is it that tells you that things are at three and not at one?'

Remember to elaborate on any of the external or internal resources described. The patient might be getting out of bed because 'well, I have to, don't I?' Asking her why she has to might reveal that she has to get up to feed the children and get them ready for school. You will be able to explore her sense of responsibility towards her children (an internal resource) further and how it shows itself and who might notice and how she feels when they do notice – remember thoughts, feelings and behaviours! Get a history of resources. Drawing the scale as in Figure 13.3 below can be helpful.

Invest lots of energy here, teasing out all those factors that may be helping already.

We can then go about exploring the characteristics of the next step on the scale:

'What will tell you that you have moved one point up the scale?'
'What would be different if you were at four instead of three?'
'What would Oscar notice about you if you were at four rather than three? . . . how would you know he had noticed? . . . What would that make you feel? . . . What would happen then? . . . So you would be feeling a little brighter and you might be going for a walk with Oscar . . . What might you be thinking about? . . . etc . . . etc . . . etc'

If the patient returns to problem-speak it is important to acknowledge the issues before gently moving back to the scale. Remember from the previous chapter the need for reflective listening. We should provide a summary statement, including some of the problem-speak, but with extra emphasis on the change material – what has been working, internal and external resources and the positive potential impact of change.

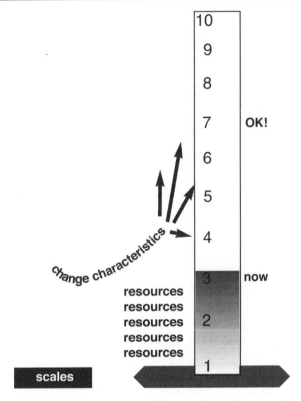

FIGURE 13.3 Scales

BOX 13.5 CASE STUDY

A lady aged 28 had low self-esteem, understandable given the abuse she suffered in childhood. She had been under the care of the psychiatric services for many years. There had been a lot of problem talk; she seemed to have a very good understanding of why she was like she was but this understanding had not helped her to feel any better. Along the way she had forgotten about past interests and achievements. All she seemed to recognise about herself was that she was a miserable 'fat blob' with scars on her forearms from her self-harming; that she was useless and had nothing to offer the world and that the world had nothing to offer her. Her view of the future was very negative.

We had discovered some of her resources that had kept her at three rather than at two on her scale. I asked her what would be happening if she was a four. She thought for a while and then told me she would be drawing again. We were able to explore when she first started drawing; what she used to draw; how it made her feel; what she thought about while she was drawing . . . etc . . . etc . . . – elaboration, elaboration, elaboration – using the thoughts-feelings-behaviours framework. Again, you could notice a change in her affect as we discussed this, with the atmosphere feeling lighter.

Change in a specific area

At this point our learning from the last chapter – **promoting change in a specific area** – can be very helpful.

She might not have been ready to jump into drawing again. We needed to explore her ambivalence about this.

> 'Your past experience of having drawing in your life sounds very positive – would it be OK if we further explored this area?'
> 'What thoughts do you have, if any, about the prospect of being involved with drawing again?'
> [*reflective listening and summarising . . .*]
> 'So, on one hand you are worried that you will not be able to draw as well as you used to . . . and on the other hand you are aware that drawing gave you a sense of achievement and it could possibly distract you from your problems and bolster your self-esteem.'

It might be helpful to employ importance and confidence scaling questions to further explore ambivalence (*see* Chapter 12).

Further open questions:

> 'Where do we go from here?'
> 'What is the next step?'
> [*Elaborate anything that she offers*]

You might have some ideas about the way forward – but ask permission before sharing them.

> 'I have some ideas about what may or may not be helpful . . . would it be OK if I shared them with you?' [*You might be aware of local resources/services that could help her to begin drawing. These might include adult education classes, local mental health projects. Voluntary sector input benefits people presenting with psychosocial problems in primary care.*[5]]

> 'Some people I have met have benefited from an art group run at the Beehive Centre. Others have found enjoyment from attending an adult education class – they have benefited from meeting some new people there. Alternatively, you might just like to try a bit of drawing alone to start with for fun. You probably

have your own ideas; after all you are the expert when it comes to knowing you. What do you think?'

'Would you be interested in learning more about how the way we think/worry about things affects the way we feel and how we can balance our thinking in a way that helps us to move forward?' [*She might be holding extreme negative beliefs about her ability to draw again and these might not be fully justified – link to self-help CBT options.*]

You could brainstorm together (*see* Chapter 12) – you might have a directory of local services, mental health or otherwise, that the patient could borrow. Remember:

> 'Who would be least surprised if you started to draw again?' (*see* Chapter 12)

You could ask if she had noticed a **vicious cycle** developing such as that described in Chapter 8.

Scales for multiple problems

When there is a whole list of problems it can be useful to have an 'overall scale' along with 'specific scales'. My patient who miraculously benefited from the 'what needs to be different?' question might have benefited from this approach.

The overall scale:

10 = everything resolved
1 = problems too overwhelming so that cannot function/cannot get out of bed

Specific scales:

➤ Never aware of pain – always crippled by severe pain
➤ Relationship harmonious all the time – extreme disharmony all the time
➤ Feeling happy all the time – never feeling happiness
➤ Spending every moment with best friend – never seeing best friend

It can be helpful to explore how a change in one area can impact on other areas:

> 'If the time spent with your friend went up one point, what effect would this have on your overall scale? . . .'

> 'What impact would it have on your awareness of pain scale?'
> etc, etc

End of session

Always give a feedback summary with affirmations.

If you have agreed the 'next step' (e.g. starting to draw again) and the way of achieving it, then state the plan and ask: *'Is that your understanding of the plan?'*

You might like to leave things as they are with a plan to meet again.

Document what you have discovered (what needs to be different, strengths and resources, point on the scale, what would characterise the next point on the scale) and any agreed task.

Putting what has been discovered in a feedback letter to the patient can be a powerful reference tool for the patient and useful documentation for us.

The next session

Beginning with a summary of the last encounter can be a good way to kick off.

> 'What has been better?'

Asking where she is on her scale now – and further use of the scale. Remember that a small change can have a knock-on effect on other areas of life.

If she says things are worse:

> 'What have you been doing that has prevented it from being even worse?'
> 'What things in your life have managed to stay OK despite going through a tough period?'

End the session with the usual summary with affirmations.

Stuart and Lieberman have developed the 'positive BATHE technique':[4]

B: 'What's the Best thing that's happened to you lately?'
One study found that asking people to list three things that went well each day and their causes increased happiness and decreased depressive symptoms over a six-month period.[6]

A: 'How do you Account for that?'

T: 'What are you most Thankful for?'
Keeping a gratitude journal has been shown to have a positive influence on physical and emotional well-being.[7]

H: 'How can you make things like that Happen more frequently?'

E': Empathy or Empowerment – 'That's exciting, I'm sure you'll do it.'

REFERENCES

1. Fairburn CG, Jones R, Peveler RC, *et al.* Three psychological treatments for bulimia nervosa. A comparative trial. *Arch Gen Psychiatry.* 1991; **48**: 463–9.
2. Fairburn CG, Jones R, Peveler RC, *et al.* Psychotherapy and bulimia nervosa. Longer-term effects of interpersonal psychotherapy, behavior therapy, and cognitive behavior therapy. *Arch Gen Psychiatry.* 1993; **50**: 419–28.
3. Agras WS, Walsh BT, Fairburn CG, *et al.* A multicenter comparison of cognitive-behavioral therapy and interpersonal psychotherapy for bulimia nervosa. *Arch Gen Psychiatry.* 2000 May; **57**: 459–66.
4. Stuart MR, Lieberman JA. *The Fifteen Minute Hour: Therapeutic Talk in Primary Care.* 4th ed. Oxford: Radcliffe Publishing; 2008.
5. Grant C, Goodenough T, Harvey I, *et al.* A randomised controlled trial and economic evaluation of a referrals facilitator between primary care and the voluntary sector. *BMJ.* 2000; **320**: 419–23.
6. Seligman MEP, Steen TA, Park N, *et al.* Positive psychology progress: empirical validation of interventions. *Am Psychol.* 2005; **60**(5): 410–21.
7. Emmons RA, McCullough ME. Counting blessings versus burdens: experimental studies of gratitude and subjective well-being in daily life. *J Pers & Soc Psychol.* 2003; **84**: 377–89.

FURTHER INFORMATION/TRAINING IN BRIEF THERAPY TECHNIQUES

➤ Stuart MR, Lieberman JA. *The Fifteen Minute Hour: Therapeutic Talk in Primary Care.* 4th ed. Oxford: Radcliffe Publishing; 2008.
   A book about incorporating useful knowledge from psychology and psychotherapy into medical practice to become more effective in dealing with the emotional overlay or underlay of the problems patients bring to the primary care practitioner.
➤ George E, Iveson C, Ratner H. *Problem to Solution: Brief Therapy with Individuals and Families.* 2nd ed. London: BT Press; 1999.
   The authors (of *The Brief Therapy Practice* – below) give a concise description of the solution-focused model. There are case studies showing the effectiveness of a solution focus with children, families and individuals with problems as diverse as depression, child protection and bulimia.
➤ The Brief Therapy Practice:
   www.brieftherapy.org.uk
   Provision of training
➤ Mark Morris Medical Ltd
   www.psychologicaltools.co.uk
   Specialising in training for general practitioners, trainee general practitioners and other primary care health professionals

➤ The Solution-Focused Brief Therapy Association
www.sfbta.org
Further resources

PART FOUR

Patient resources

Advice for problem drinking

HAVE TWO NON-ALCOHOL DRINKING DAYS/WEEK

Who?	How many drinks?	How often?
Men	No more than three units	Each day (only for five days/week)
Women	No more than two units	Each day (only for five days/week)

RECOMMENDATION IS NOT TO DRINK IN THE FOLLOWING SITUATIONS

➤ Pregnancy.
➤ Physical alcohol dependence.
➤ Physical problems made worse by drinking.
➤ Driving, biking.
➤ Operating machinery.
➤ Exercising (swimming, jogging, etc).

HOW TO REACH TARGET LEVELS

➤ Keep track of your alcohol consumption.
➤ Turn to family and/or friends for support.
➤ Have one or more non-alcoholic drinks before each drink.
➤ Delay the time of day that you drink.
➤ Take smaller sips.
➤ Switch to low-alcohol drinks.
➤ Decide on non-drinking days (two days or more per week).

➤ Eat before starting to drink.
➤ Join a support group.
➤ Quench your thirst with non-alcoholic drinks.

Remember the cue issue:
➤ Engage in alternative activities at times that you would normally drink (e.g. when you are feeling bored or stressed).
➤ Avoid or reduce time spent with heavy-drinking friends.
➤ Avoid bars, cafes or former drinking places.

REVIEW PROGRESS: ARE YOU KEEPING ON TRACK? PROGRESS TIPS

➤ Every week record how much you drink over the week.
➤ Avoid these difficult situations or plan activities to help you cope with them.
➤ Think back to your original reasons for cutting down or stopping.
➤ Come back for help, talk to family and friends.

Patient resources: anxiety biology

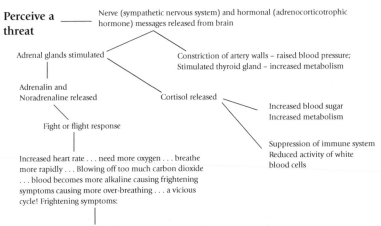

Perceive a ———— Nerve (sympathetic nervous system) and hormonal (adrenocorticotrophic
threat hormone) messages released from brain

Adrenal glands stimulated

Constriction of artery walls – raised blood pressure;
Stimulated thyroid gland – increased metabolism

Adrenalin and
Noradrenaline released

Cortisol released

Increased blood sugar
Increased metabolism

Fight or flight response

Suppression of immune system
Reduced activity of white
blood cells

Increased heart rate . . . need more oxygen . . . breathe
more rapidly . . . Blowing off too much carbon dioxide
. . . blood becomes more alkaline causing frightening
symptoms causing more over-breathing . . . a vicious
cycle! Frightening symptoms:

**Tight chest; Rapid heartbeat; Sweating; Tingling; Feeling faint;
Feeling of unreality; Blurred vision; Rigid muscles; Feeling too hot/
too cold; Muscles of anus and bladder relax . . . want to use the toilet
(it is best to be as light as possible when a lion is chasing you!)**

Safer injecting

> Always inject in the direction of blood flow and position the needle with the long side nearest to the skin, with the needle at a 10- to 20-degree angle to the skin.
> Always use a clean needle and syringe with each drug injection.
> Rotate injecting sites, preferably in the arms.
> Use smallest bore needle possible.
> Use light, warmth, and clenching and re-clenching the fist to make seeing and accessing the vein easier.
> Try to avoid use of tourniquets – this raises the venous pressure, making blood leakage and subsequent damage more likely.
> If blood appears in the barrel very quickly, is bright red, injection is particularly painful, or requires undue pressure, do not continue with the injection as these are the signs of arterial injection (this is particularly important advice for groin injectors).
> Apply pressure to the site for at least 30 seconds after injection to prevent blood leakage and subsequent damage.
> Avoid injecting into the neck or groin.
> Try to avoid injecting into the veins of the breast, feet and hands.
> Avoid tablet injecting, as tablets often contain large quantities of insoluble material.
> If crushing tablets filter, solution before injecting.
> Always dispose of your equipment safely (either in a bin provided by the needle exchange or by placing your used needle inside the syringe and placing both inside a drinks can and dispose of the can appropriately).
> Never inject into infected areas.
> Do not inject into swollen limbs even if the veins appear to be distended.
> Don't inject drugs alone – this is a known risk factor for fatal overdose.

➤ Don't inject others.
➤ Keep others safe, spread these messages to other injectors, and don't initiate others to injecting.

Disordered eating: the risks and self-help

This information is taken from www.eatingresearch.com, the eating disorder information website from the Institute of Psychiatry. This site is packed with very useful information for you and for those close to you. Other useful resources are listed at the end of this information.

There are three categories of behaviour that pose a risk.
1 Starvation and restriction of food.
2 Purging.
3 Binge-eating episodes.

Although a person might be suffering specifically with anorexia, bulimia or binge-eating disorder, it is possible that she or he might exhibit behaviours from each of the three. It is also not uncommon for one eating disorder to be swapped for another (e.g. a person with anorexia switches to bulimia; a person with compulsive overeating switches to anorexia).

THE EFFECTS OF STARVATION

➤ Sensitivity to cold: poor circulation results in hands and feet becoming blue, mottled, swollen and subject to chilblains. Some women with anorexia have died of hypothermia.
➤ Sleep disturbances: waking up early or several times in the night.
➤ Weak bladder: passing water frequently throughout the day or night.
➤ Lanugo: excess hair growth on the body, particularly on the back and the sides of the face. This is caused by a built-in protective mechanism to help keep a person warm during periods of starvation and malnutrition and the hormonal imbalances that result.

➤ Muscle atrophy: wasting away of muscle and decrease in muscle mass due to the body feeding off itself.

➤ Poor circulation, slow pulse, low blood pressure and fainting spells.

➤ Osteoporosis: the progressive thinning of bones, resulting from calcium, magnesium and/or vitamin D deficiency may result in fracture leading to deformity and pain. Hormone imbalance associated with the loss of the menstrual cycle can also increase the risk of osteoporosis.

➤ Menstrual irregularities: periods stop or become very irregular. It is usually only possible for a woman to have periods when 15% of her body is composed of fat. Malnutrition and vitamin deficiencies can also make it impossible to succeed with a full-term pregnancy, and can significantly increase the chances of a baby born with birth defects.

➤ Loss of libido: in anorexia the sexual organs shrink in size and structure to those of a child before puberty. Without the hormonal environment associated with maturity the sexual drive disappears. This occurs in both women and men.

➤ Stomach shrinkage: The stomach shrinks and feels uncomfortably distended after eating even a small amount of food. Stomach ulcers may be a problem that persists after recovery.

➤ Constipation: as a result of the slow-down of gut function.

➤ The bone marrow fails: red and white blood cells are not formed quickly enough which results in anaemia and susceptibility to certain infections.

➤ Liver: the lack of nutrition affects the liver so that it is unable to manufacture body proteins. This may result in swelling of the ankles and legs.

➤ Blood cholesterol is increased: this results from the lack of oestrogen (before the menopause women are protected from heart attacks by oestrogen).

➤ Nerves and muscles become damaged: this may make it difficult to climb stairs, the feet may drag and extreme fatigue and tiredness results. Left untreated, periods of paralysis may occur, leading to permanent muscle weakness.

➤ Growth may be stunted and puberty delayed in younger children.

➤ Low glucose: this produces feelings of panic or light-headedness. If ignored, it can lead to coma and death.

➤ Dehydration: caused by lack of intake of fluids or by restriction of carbohydrates and fat. Symptoms include dizziness, weakness or darkening of the urine. It can lead to kidney failure, heart failure, seizures, brain damage and death.

➤ Hyponatremia: drinking too much water (more than eight 8 oz glasses in less than 12 hours) can cause a depletion of sodium in the blood, especially in someone already malnourished or dehydrated. This can cause fluid in the lungs, nausea, vomiting, confusion, brain swelling and even death.

➤ Dry skin and hair, brittle nails, hair loss: caused by vitamin and mineral deficiencies, malnutrition and dehydration.

➤ Easily bruising skin: vitamin deficiencies that decrease the body's ability to heal itself, low blood pressure, low platelet count and/or extreme weight loss all lead to easily bruised skin that can take a long time to heal.

➤ 'I felt drained, tired, lonely, hungry, in despair, tired legs, constipated, very cold and was anaemic'.

THE EFFECTS OF VOMITING, LAXATIVE AND DIURETIC USE

➤ Electrolyte imbalances: water and salt imbalances may disturb the function of the heart, brain and kidneys. Potassium levels can become very low and disturb the electrical activity of the heart and brain, leading to heart attacks and fits.

➤ Oedema: swelling of the soft tissues as a result of excess water accumulation can be caused by laxative and diuretic use.

➤ Tearing of the oesophagus: caused by self-induced vomiting.

➤ Mallory-Weiss tear: a tear of the gastro-oesophageal junction, associated with vomiting.

➤ Gastric rupture: spontaneous stomach erosion, perforation or rupture.

➤ Gastro-intestinal bleeding: bleeding into the digestive tract.

➤ Oesophageal reflux: acid reflux disorders – partially digested items in the stomach, mixed with acid and enzymes, regurgitate back into the oesophagus. This can lead to damage to the oesophagus, larynx and lungs and increases the chances of developing cancer of the oesophagus and the larynx.

➤ Swelling of the salivary glands: in the face and cheeks following self-induced vomiting.

➤ Callused or bruised fingers: this is caused by repeated use of the fingers to induce vomiting.

➤ Disruptions in blood sugar levels: low blood sugar (hypoglycaemia) can lead to neurological and mental deterioration. High blood sugar (hypoglycaemia) can lead to diabetes, liver and kidney shut-down, circulatory and immune system problems.

➤ Ketoacidosis: high levels of acids that build up in the blood (known as ketones) caused by the body burning fat instead of sugar and carbohydrates to get energy. It can be the result of starvation, excessive purging, dehydration, hyperglycaemia and/or alcohol abuse, and it can lead to coma and death.

➤ Dental problems: including decalcification of teeth, erosion of tooth enamel, severe decay and gum disease are caused by stomach acids and enzymes from vomiting; vitamin D and calcium deficiencies and hormonal imbalance.

➤ Menstrual problems: as mentioned above.

➤ Digestive problems: including constipation, diarrhoea, incontinence, peptic ulcers. A deficiency in digestive enzymes will lead to the body's inability to properly digest food and absorb nutrients. A history of eating disorders can sometimes trigger celiac disease (gluten sensitivity) and Crohn's disease.

➤ Pancreatitis: this occurs when the digestive enzymes attack the pancreas. It can be caused by repeated stomach trauma (such as with vomiting), alcohol consumption or the excessive use of laxatives or diet pills.

➤ Arthritis: this can be caused by hormonal imbalances and vitamin deficiencies as well as increased stress on the joints in individuals with binge-eating disorder or who over-exercise.

EFFECTS OF OVER-EXERCISE

➤ Low blood sugar: when this is very low, it can lead to coma and even death.

➤ Stress fractures: as the bones are thin, stress fractures emerge.

➤ Damage to muscles and joints: in the context of starvation, over-exercise destroys muscle as the body consumes its own flesh. Damage to joints can cause arthritis in the long term.

EFFECTS OF BINGEING

➤ Obesity: common among individuals with binge-eating disorder, but the relationship between binge-eating and obesity is far from clear.

➤ Diabetes: this is more likely to occur in overweight individuals, but can also occur as a result of hormonal imbalances, hyperglycemia or chronic pancreatitis.

➤ Arthritis: increased stress on the joints in individuals with binge-eating disorder can lead to arthritis in the long term.

CAN EATING DISORDERS CAUSE PERMANENT DAMAGE?

It is difficult to answer this with confidence, as there have been relatively few studies which have followed the health of sufferers over time.

Most of the physical problems do reverse with weight gain, or if the weight control practices stop. It may depend on the duration of the illness and the stage of life at which the illness arose. For example, there may be a critical time at which puberty can take place. If the illness strikes before all stages of puberty have been attained and recovery is delayed, there may be irreversible failure to achieve growth in stature, peak bone density and secondary sexual development.

Adolescence is also a critical period for cognitive and psychosocial develop-ment, and it is simply not known whether an individual will be able to reach their full potential in cognitive and psychosocial development if they recover after this critical period has passed.

It is probable that, if there is full recovery, all will return to normal with the reproductive system, although it may take longer than normal to conceive. In some cases, it may be necessary to have hormonal treatment. The difficulty is that between one-third and one-half of all sufferers may have residual problems and are still under their optimal weight.

We do not know by how much bone density recovers. There is some evidence that with a short illness the bones can regain their strength and thickness. It may take a long time for the repairs to be completed and some sites are repaired before others. Recovery may be incomplete. If the bones remain thin, the risk of fracture is increased. Bones in the spinal column may be crushed, and the spinal curvature and subsequent loss of height are irreversible. This may lead to chronic pain.

In the general population 'yo-yo' dieting is associated with an increased risk of cardiovascular disease and death. Patients on very low fat diets often have raised levels of cholesterol, which may be a risk factor for heart disease.

After recovery intestinal problems may remain. Heartburn and stomach ulcers are more common. The bowel can become 'irritable' with frequent diarrhoea or severe constipation.

Weight control measures that alter salt and water balance can lead to permanent kidney damage. As the kidneys have a lot of reserve function this may not become apparent unless they are put under further stress.

TIME AND LOST OPPORTUNITIES

Whatever the long-term damage to physical health, the one thing that can never be recovered is lost time. Individuals who overcome eating disorders after a number of years often express great sadness for all the missed opportunities, as illustrated by the following quotations.

'Recovery for me involved grieving for past pain and for time spent not allowing myself to be happy.'

'I find myself yearning for the teenage years I missed out on completely. Sometimes the pain is so great, it stops me enjoying to the full the good things I have gained since recovery. And then I realise what I am doing, and force myself to return to the present before I lose any more time!'

SELF-HELP RESOURCES
Books
Anorexia nervosa
Anorexia Nervosa: A Survival Guide for Families, Friends and Sufferers
Janet Treasure
Psychology Press 1997
ISBN 0-86377-760-0

When anorexia nervosa strikes an individual and their family, everyone is thrown into confusion. This book attempts to answer some of the questions that are asked by everyone.

'At this point in my life I am struggling to keep my weight high enough to stay out of hospital. This book made the risks I am running clear to me as well as providing me with helpful ideas about how to conquer this awful illness. I am a long way from recovery but this book has definitely made a huge impression on me and is the only one I have read that has helped.'

'This great book (and I have read many) is a clearly written, practical guide for sufferers and their families. Unlike some, the focus here is more on the signs that anorexia is affecting someone and the practical steps one can take to recover from it rather than an over-emphasis on the deep psychological causes. THE Anorexia bible. I wouldn't be without it.'

Bulimia nervosa and binge-eating disorders
Getting Better Bit(e) by Bit(e): A Survival Kit for Sufferers of Bulimia Nervosa and Binge-Eating Disorders
Ulrike Schmidt, Janet Treasure
Psychology Press 1993
ISBN 0-86377-322-2

This self-help book, whose efficacy has been proven in clinical trials, empowers sufferers to take control of their own lives and tackle their eating difficulties in their own home.

> 'This book is easy to follow. You can either read it all in one go or dip into it whenever you feel like it. I would suggest it to everyone who is trying to get help for an eating disorder and (as in my case) those who have received the help and are tentatively trying life out without the support of a counsellor any more. It provides that bit of support when you're feeling wobbly and helps you to continue to move forward with the confidence that you aren't alone.'

Online

Eating Disorders Association: http://new.edauk.com/
This is a nationwide organisation that offers a number of services including telephone advice, self-help groups, family groups and individual counselling, training courses and information on service provision.

Eating disorder information website from the Institute of Psychiatry: www.eatingresearch.com
A wealth of helpful information.

Appendices

Alcohol questionnaires

AUDIT – C

1 How often have you had a drink containing alcohol in the past year?

Never	0
Monthly or less	1
2–4 times per month	2
2–3 times per week	3
4 or more times per week	4

2 How many alcoholic drinks do you have on a typical day when you are drinking?

1 or 2	0
3 or 4	1
5 or 6	2
7 to 10	3
10 or more	4

3 How often do you have six drinks or more on one occasion?

Never	0
Less than monthly	1
Monthly	2
Weekly	3
Daily or almost daily	4

➤ Score suggestive of hazardous drinking = 8 or more. Consider use of the CAGE questionnaire below to help identify alcohol dependence.
➤ In men scoring 4–7 and women scoring 3–7 consider advice and brief intervention [*see* FRAMES in Chapter 5].
➤ If all the points scored come from Q1 then confirm that this pattern is long-standing – 'Has this been your consistent pattern of drinking over the last three months?' If so, no need for concern.

Bush K, Kivlahan DR, McDonell, *et al.* The AUDIT alcohol consumption questions (AUDIT-C): an effective brief screening test for problem drinking. *Arch Intern Med.* 1998; 158: 1789–95.

CAGE QUESTIONNAIRE

Alcohol dependence is likely if the patient gives two or more positive answers to the following questions.
➤ Have you ever felt you should **Cut** down on your drinking?
➤ Have people **Annoyed** you by criticising your drinking?
➤ Have you ever felt bad or **Guilty** about your drinking?
➤ Have you ever had a drink first thing in the morning to steady your nerves or get rid of a hangover (an eye-opener)?

Ewing JA. Detecting alcoholism. The CAGE questionnaire. *JAMA.* 1984; 252(14): 1905–7.

Edinburgh Postnatal Depression Scale Questionnaire

As you have recently had a baby, we would like to know how you are feeling now. Please UNDERLINE the answer which comes closest to how you have felt in THE PAST SEVEN DAYS, not just how you feel today.

Here is an example already completed:

I have felt happy:

Yes, most of the time

Yes, some of the time

No, not very often

No, not at all

This would mean: 'I have felt happy some of the time' during the past week.

Please complete the other questions in the same way.

1 I have been able to laugh and see the funny side of things:

As much as I always could	0
Not quite so much now	1
Definitely not so much now	2
Not at all	3

2 I have looked forward with enjoyment to things:

As much as I ever did	0
Rather less than I used to	1
Definitely less that I used to	2
Hardly at all	3

3 I have blamed myself unnecessarily when things went wrong:

Yes, most of the time	3
Yes, some of the time	2
Not very often	1
No, never	0

4 I have felt worried or anxious for no very good reason:

No, not at all	0
Hardly ever	1
Yes, sometimes	2
Yes, very often	3

5 I have felt scared or panicky for no very good reason:

Yes, quite a lot	3
Yes, sometimes	2
No, not much	1
No, not at all	0

6 Things have been getting on top of me:

Yes, most of the time I haven't been able to cope at all	3
Yes, sometimes I haven't been coping as well as usual	2
No, most of the time I have coped quite well	1
No, I have been coping as well as ever	0

7 I have been so unhappy that I have had difficulty sleeping:

Yes, most of the time	3
Yes, sometimes	2
Not very often	1
No, not at all	0

8 I have felt sad or miserable:

Yes, most of the time	3
Yes, quite often	2
Not very often	1
No, not at all	0

9 I have been so unhappy that I have been crying:

Yes, most of the time	3
Yes, quite often	2
Only occasionally	1
No, never	0

10 The thought of harming myself has occurred to me:

Yes, quite often	3
Sometimes	2
Hardly ever	1
Never	0

Cox JL, Holden JN, Sagovsky R. Detection of postnatal depression: development of the 10-item Edinburgh Postnatal Depression Scale. *Br J Psychiatry.* 1987; 150: 782–6.

Mini mental state examination

Mini mental state examination	
Orientation in time Can you tell me today's (date), (month), and (year)? Which (day) is it today? Which (season) is it?	5
Orientation in place What town are we in? What is the (county)/(country)? What (building) are we in and on what (floor)?	5
Registration Name three common objects: for example, ball, car, and man Can you repeat the words I said? (score one point for each word)	3
Attention and calculation Subtract seven from 100. Stop after five answers. (93, 86, 79, 72, 65) *Alternatively* Spell the word 'world' backwards. (d, l, r, o, w)	5
Recall What were the three words I asked you to say earlier? (*Skip this test if all three objects were not remembered during the registration test*).	3
Naming Name these objects. (show a watch and a pencil)	2

Repeating Repeat the following: 'no ifs ands or buts'	1
Reading Write *'Close your eyes'* on a card. Read this sentence and do what it says.	1
Writing Can you write a short sentence for me?	1
Language: three-stage command Take this piece of paper in your left hand, fold it in half and put it on the floor.	3

Construction
Copy this drawing please.

1

Total score (out of 30)

Folstein MF, Folstein SE, McHugh PR. 'Mini-mental state'. A practical method for grading the cognitive state of patients for the clinician. *J Psychiatr Res.* 1975; 12(3): 189–98.

BMI Centile charts

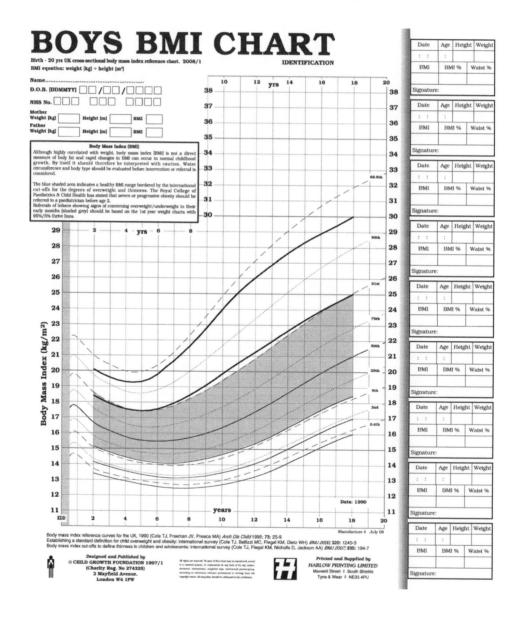

GIRLS BMI CHART

Birth - 20 yrs UK cross-sectional body mass index reference chart. 2008/1

BMI equation: weight [kg] ÷ height [m²]

IDENTIFICATION

Name...

D.O.B. [DDMMYY] ☐☐ / ☐☐ / ☐☐☐☐

NHS No. ☐☐☐   ☐☐☐   ☐☐☐☐

Mother
Weight [kg] ☐   Height [m] ☐   BMI ☐

Father
Weight [kg] ☐   Height [m] ☐   BMI ☐

Body Mass Index (BMI)

Although highly correlated with weight, body mass index [BMI] is not a direct measure of body fat and rapid changes in BMI can occur in normal childhood growth. By itself it should therefore be interpreted with caution. Waist circumference and body type should be evaluated before intervention or referral is considered.

The blue shaded area indicates a healthy BMI range bordered by the international cut-offs for the degrees of overweight and thinness. The Royal College of Paediatrics & Child Health has stated that severe or progressive obesity should be referred to a paediatrician before age 2.

Referrals of infants showing signs of concerning overweight/underweight in their early months [shaded grey] should be based on the 1st year weight charts with 95%/5% thrive lines.

Body Mass Index (kg/m²)

Data: 1990

Manufacture 4   July 08

Body mass index reference curves for the UK, 1990 (Cole TJ, Freeman JV, Preece MA) *Arch Dis Child* 1995; 73: 25-9
Establishing a standard definition for child overweight and obesity: international survey (Cole TJ, Bellizzi MC, Flegal KM, Dietz WH) *BMJ 2000*; **320**: 1240-3
Body mass index cut-offs to define thinness in children and adolescents: international survey (Cole TJ, Flegal KM, Nicholls D, Jackson AA) *BMJ 2007*; **335**: 194-7

Designed and Published by
© **CHILD GROWTH FOUNDATION 1997/1**
(Charity Reg. No 274325)
2 Mayfield Avenue,
London W4 1PW

Printed and Supplied by
HARLOW PRINTING LIMITED
Maxwell Street ◊ South Shields
Tyne & Wear ◊ NE33 4PU

Date	Age	Height	Weight
: :	:		
BMI	BMI %		Waist %
Signature:			

Date	Age	Height	Weight
: :	:		
BMI	BMI %		Waist %
Signature:			

Date	Age	Height	Weight
: :	:		
BMI	BMI %		Waist %
Signature:			

Date	Age	Height	Weight
: :	:		
BMI	BMI %		Waist %
Signature:			

Date	Age	Height	Weight
: :	:		
BMI	BMI %		Waist %
Signature:			

Date	Age	Height	Weight
: :	:		
BMI	BMI %		Waist %
Signature:			

Date	Age	Height	Weight
: :	:		
BMI	BMI %		Waist %
Signature:			

Date	Age	Height	Weight
: :	:		
BMI	BMI %		Waist %
Signature:			

Date	Age	Height	Weight
: :	:		
BMI	BMI %		Waist %
Signature:			

Index